Statistical Reasoning for Surgeons

Statistical Reasoning
for Surgeons

Mitchell G. Maltenfort
Camilo Restrepo
Antonia F. Chen

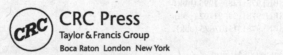

CRC Press
Taylor & Francis Group
Boca Raton London New York

CRC Press is an imprint of the
Taylor & Francis Group, an **informa** business

A CHAPMAN & HALL BOOK

First edition published 2021
by CRC Press
6000 Broken Sound Parkway NW, Suite 300, Boca Raton, FL 33487-2742

and by CRC Press
2 Park Square, Milton Park, Abingdon, Oxon, OX14 4RN

ISBN: 9781138091795 (hbk)
ISBN: 9781138091702 (pbk)
ISBN: 9781315107875 (ebk)

Typeset in Minion
by Deanta Global Publishing Services, Chennai, India

Access the Support Material: www.routledge.com/9781138091702

To my father Lee Maltenfort who taught me wit and brevity,
and to my grandfather Paul who taught him

Contents

Preface, xi

Authors' Biographies, xiii

CHAPTER 1 ■ Introduction – Why Does a Surgeon
Need Statistics?   1

CHAPTER 2 ■ Interpreting Probability: Medical
School Axioms of Probability   11

HORSES BEFORE ZEBRAS   17

THE SIMPLEST EXPLANATION IS MOST LIKELY   19

THE PATIENT CAN HAVE AS MANY DISEASES AS
THEY PLEASE   19

THERE ARE MORE DIFFERENCES BETWEEN BAD
MEDICINE AND GOOD MEDICINE; THAN THERE
IS BETWEEN GOOD MEDICINE AND NO MEDICINE   20

CHAPTER 3 ■ Statistics, the Law of Large Numbers,
and the Confidence Interval   21

CHAPTER 4 ■ The Basics of Statistical Tests   29

CARE AND FEEDING OF p-VALUES   29

THE PERILS OF PRODUCTIVITY   33

SAMPLE SIZE VERSUS p-VALUES   35

ALWAYS INCLUDE THE CONFIDENCE INTERVAL   36

Chapter 5 ▪ How Much Data Is Enough? 39

Chapter 6 ▪ Showing the Data to Yourself First –
Graphs and Tables, Part 1 47

Chapter 7 ▪ How Normal Is a Gaussian
Distribution? What to Do with
Extreme Values? 55

NON-GAUSSIAN DISTRIBUTIONS 55
EXTREME VALUES 57
ORDINAL DATA 60

Chapter 8 ▪ All Probabilities Are Conditional 63

Chapter 9 ▪ Quality versus Quantity in Data 67

KNOW WHAT YOU'RE GETTING 67
PROPER LAYOUT 68
TO CATEGORIZE OR NOT TO CATEGORIZE 71

Chapter 10 ▪ Practical Examples 75

EXAMPLE 1: BLOOD LOSS 75
EXAMPLE 2: COMORBIDITIES AND MORTALITY 77
EXAMPLE 3: MINIMAL CLINICALLY IMPORTANT
DIFFERENCE 78
EXAMPLE 4: THE PARTICULAR PROBLEM OF BMI 79

Chapter 11 ▪ All Things Being Equal – But How?
(Designing the Study) 81

RANDOM ASSIGNMENT IS NOT ALWAYS AN
OPTION 81
MATCHING AND STRATIFICATION 83

SELECTING MULTIPLE PREDICTORS 83

PROPENSITY SCORES 93

ALSO CONSIDER 94

CHAPTER 12 ■ Binary and Count Outcomes 97

CHAPTER 13 ■ Repeated Measurements and
Accounting for Change 101

CHAPTER 14 ■ What If the Data Is Not All There? 107

CHAPTER 15 ■ Showing the Data to Others – Graphs
and Tables, Part 2 111

ORGANIZING THE PRESENTATION 111

PRESENTING THE NARRATIVE 112

KEEPING NUMBERS IN CONTEXT 113

TABLES VERSUS GRAPHS: SCALE AND STYLE 116

ARTICULATING THE STORY 117

VISUAL LINGO 118

CHAPTER 16 ■ Further Reading 121

GLOSSARY, 125

REFERENCES, 129

INDEX, 135

Preface

THE PARTICULAR CHALLENGE OF clinical research is that effective clinicians and effective researchers each exploit different modes of intelligence. The clinician has to think of the body as a coordinated whole, in which different organs may interact directly or indirectly with each other and with various physical factors such as injury, toxins, infection, or medical intervention. The researcher has to take a reductionist and quantitative view, looking at what can be measured or calculated and comparing observed facts against speculation. Perspectives, too, are different: a clinician will see a patient as an individual case with a history and a trajectory, which may or may not overlap with similar cases, while in research data has to be seen in the aggregate and the abstract.

There's an old joke about a farmer who hires scientists to figure out ways to improve milk production. The first line of the report is "consider a spherical cow." The punchline is the frequent disconnect between the physical world and the mathematical one.

Statistics can be seen as an attempt to make the connection, using mathematical tools to analyze measurable variables and distill useful information. This is necessarily limited. A quote attributed to Albert Einstein is 'Not everything that can be counted counts and not everything that counts can be counted.' We can tally days in the hospital, the number of infections, and so on. There are no distinct physical units for pain or suffering, and patient-reported outcome measures are only an approximate measure. But the effort is justified when the results lead to an improvement in patient care.

This book began in the traditional literary manner as a way to let off steam. Clinical research is frustrating for many reasons. However, it can also be rewarding. While the astute reader will catch us in several places venting over our own issues, the main motivation (we insist!) is to help other researchers avoid the frustrations and have a better chance of the rewards.

Authors' Biographies

Mitchell G. Maltenfort lurched into academic life as a computational neurobiologist before drifting into the less recherché field of biostatistics. He knows just enough to make a complete hash out of things and is creative enough to salvage them afterward. In his brutish culture, this tradition is known as "larnin." For tax purposes, he is employed as a biostatistician at Children's Hospital of Philadelphia, where he has generated risk scores for hospitalization; analyzed diagnostic variations among clinics; compared international trends in childhood mortality; and evaluated patient-reported outcome scores.

Camilo Restrepo is the Associate Director for Research at the Rothman Institute (RI), Philadelphia, PA. He is known informally at RI as "Doctor Data."

Antonia F. Chen is the Director of Research for Arthroplasty Services at Brigham and Women's Hospital and an Associate Professor at Harvard Medical School, Boston, MA. She is a past president of the Musculoskeletal Infection Society (MSIS) and is an active collaborator in research studies on topics including infection outcomes and opioid use. She often travels armed with a small and extremely cute dog named Lily, who is often the highlight of research meetings where Lily is in attendance.

CHAPTER 1

Introduction – Why Does a Surgeon Need Statistics?

Patients considering surgery will ask what their future would be, with or without surgery. Will symptoms get better or worse, and by how much? What measures can they take to improve things, and how much good will that do? What complications might they face if they had surgery, and how likely are those complications? When something goes wrong, they – or their families or lawyers – will demand to know whether it could have been foreseen.

The surgeon, of course, wants to be able to provide useful and insightful answers. These answers will probably be from published journal articles or textbooks based on published articles and so will usually be in the form of statistics. Surgeons may also need to answer for themselves what complication rates to expect or what they can do to improve their outcomes across their practice. This also scales up; hospitals will have departments with multiple surgeons, and insurers will cover patients seen at multiple hospitals.

Statements like "this procedure has a 2% complication rate for patients," "having a specific condition makes your risk of problems three times greater," or "the average patient recovers within three months" are essentially weather forecasts that provide a description of probability based on (presumably) careful analyses of data, although the consequences may be more severe than just getting caught in the rain. The problem is, how reliable is a weather forecast? Temperature and humidity numbers never seem off by much, but the chance of rain never seems tightly associated with when the clouds decide to open.

In practice, we do not want to predict outcomes or complications like we would want to predict the weather. We want to prevent complications and ensure good outcomes. Falling short of that level of perfect control, we want to identify what situations are associated with good and bad outcomes, so we can make better choices. The individual patient wants the best chances at a satisfactory outcome. The surgeon, who sees many patients, wants to show a consistent pattern of success. Hospitals and insurance companies would like to avoid the costs associated with procedures that do not benefit patients and reduce the likelihood of complications such as readmissions and reoperations. This balancing act tries to ensure that the best possible care is offered to the largest number of patients while anticipating that inevitable fraction proving the surgical adage: "You officially become a surgeon when you do everything right and the patient still has problems."

One of the subtleties of statistics is that you can use the same tools to ask different questions. For example, say you did a statistical analysis looking at how patient factors predict surgical complications. Some of these are adjustable, such as weight and smoking, and so the surgeon could say to the patient that changing these habits can improve outcomes by such-and-such an amount. Some are not, such as age or diagnosis, but then the model could still be used to estimate the overall complication risk and perhaps determine which patients have unacceptably high risks. The surgeon might also discover that a particular way of doing surgery is doing more harm than good – or not doing any good at all – and so select an alternative approach that is better for the patient or that doesn't waste time or resources for no real benefit.

Certain aphorisms learned in medical school are actually applicable to doing statistics:

- Look for horses before zebras (look for common things before rare things).

- The simplest explanation is the most likely to be true.

- The patient can have as many diseases as they please.

- There are more differences between bad medicine and good medicine; then there is between good medicine and no medicine.

Each of these proverbs describes how probability affects patient outcomes, although they may not seem relevant to the formulas taught in statistics class. As with any field, it can take practical experience to fully appreciate the connections between classroom instruction and real-world applications.

This book is intended to help expedite this learning process by sharing lessons learned from our own varied and colorful experiences in clinical research. Part of that is bridging the gap between formal academic writing and more grounded discussion. The statement "we are designing a prognostic study to estimate the odds ratio of patient factors on outcome" is more technical but perhaps less useful than the statement "if we know how these factors affect the outcome, we can better decide which patients we can safely operate on, and make choices to better serve those patients we do operate on." There is a famous example in writing, from the British novelist Sir Arthur Quiller-Couch: the statements "he was conveyed to his place of residence in an intoxicated condition" and "he was carried home drunk" both carry the same information, but only one could be called plain language. We aspire to plain language here. You may have to move in the other direction when you prepare your manuscripts for submission, but that is between you and the journal.

We assume you have already been through some statistics instruction and have one of the many fine statistics texts out there. This book is intended to be a companion to such texts. Medicine and statistics are each too broad for us to promise you a clear path for getting from a clinical problem to a defined research question to a solid statistical analysis plan, but we can help you on the way and give some pointers on how to interpret the statistical results. We will only be getting into mathematics as necessary to clarify certain points. Regarding the clarity of statistical terms, we know that the terminology is sometimes awful. Even statisticians working in the same area will disagree about what specific terms mean. Where we define a term here, we are not being definitive or authoritative but trying to help bring some intuitive context. If, concomitant with or consequent to reading this book, you are interested in some more depth, we would recommend the course notes and lectures provided by the University of Vanderbilt online at https://hbiostat. org/bbr/ [1].

This book is in the spirit of other texts, not necessarily technical, showing the essential concepts underlying the application and presentation of statistical analysis. A favorite is Robert Abelson's *Statistics as Principled Argument* [2], which presents statistical reasoning from the perspective of how statements made can be supported or weakened. Also excellent is Stephen Stigler's *The Seven Pillars of Statistical Wisdom* [3], which examines statistics from the perspective of fundamental ideas. There are also good texts describing how statistics can be misapplied or misinterpreted by people who think they are doing it right, such as the accessible and whimsical *Statistics Done Wrong* [4] and *How to Lie with Statistics* [5], but we are considering issues more specific to clinical studies. *Common Errors in Statistics (and How to Avoid Them)* [6] is also a good, if more technical and perhaps more opinionated, book and has an excellent piece of advice: have study plans reviewed by a computer programmer or someone who writes a lot of computer code (not necessarily a statistician or a data scientist) in order to spot ambiguity and logical gaps.

This is less a "cookbook" and more of a compendium of kitchen tips for getting the most out of recipes. We want to encourage the reader to expand beyond the usual automatic approaches in statistical analyses while keeping aware of practical limitations. The principles of statistical analysis are in flux and open to debate, even among statisticians. This has been the case since the 1930s, when p-values and significance testing were first introduced and the first arguments ensued. Over the years, our approach has been to balance technical accuracy and intuitive clarity.

In this book, we will briefly describe the assumptions that are made to simplify statistical tests, whether violating the assumptions can actually cause trouble, and when you may need to present your results with warnings or consider alternative approaches that will be more appropriate to your research question. It is impractical for us to provide a completely comprehensive review of all potential situations, but the range that we do address should provide insights useful to your own research projects going forward.

As a general piece of advice, where there is concern over which approach is .best, running it each way will often be faster than debating the issues. This is a no-lose proposition. If the different approaches agree, you have strengthened your story by adding evidence (technically known as a "sensitivity analysis"). If the approaches disagree, you can add detail to your story by investigating why the results differ. No single analysis will ever be completely definitive. In a seminal 1962 paper considering the history and trajectory of statistics [7], the statistician John Tukey recommended as

the most important maxim for data analysts to heed. ...
"Far better an approximate answer to the *right* question,
which is often vague, than an *exact* answer to the wrong
question, which can always be made precise." Data analysis must progress by approximate answers ... since the
knowledge of what the problem really is will at best be
approximate.

We can never be perfect, but we can always discover ways to
improve.

Tukey also gives us caution [8]: "The combination of some
data and the aching desire for an answer does not ensure that a
reasonable answer can be extracted from a given body of data."
You're familiar with this in the general sense from the observation that years of effort from many people on a single problem
may not return satisfactory solutions. Keep this in mind for your
personal case, where you are analyzing data and trying to find a
publishable result. There may not be one, or if it seems publishable, it still may not be reliable.

Many readers will have access to Excel (or a free alternative such as OpenOffice or LibreOffice). Although Excel does
offer convenient tools for creating and formatting tables and
graphics, and we've taken advantage of those ourselves in
creating the figures for this book, serious statistical analysis
requires more sophisticated and powerful tools such as those
provided by SAS®, SPSS®, Stata®, or R®. *Data Smart* by J.W.
Foreman [9], an excellent book, describes how to use Excel®'s
optimizer for analyses ranging from logistic regression to
cluster analysis and does so in a manner that makes each of
these analyses intuitive, but the last chapter (sorry to spoil the
ending, Mr. Foreman!) recommends installing R® for readers
wanting to best apply the methods that Excel® was used to
demonstrate.

While we're in the neighborhood, we should specify that there are points in this book where we say the issues raised are tricky enough that you should discuss them with an experienced statistician. This is not to say you should not try analyzing it yourself. Go right ahead; data doesn't burn up with use, and exploring the data is recommended. But don't be shy about asking available experts for help, even if it's just to say, "I think I have this right but I wanted to check." This is one of the rare occasions that we can speak for most statisticians and state they will probably be delighted to discuss your question.

This book is divided into four sections, going from the general to the specific:

1. *Fundamental concepts and how they are applied in research.* For example, what does a 5% probability really mean? What is an average, a standard deviation (SD), or a p-value really telling us? Why do we want a minimum sample size? Do we want a statistical test or an estimated value? Frank Harrell pointed out it is one thing to estimate the probability of rain and another thing to decide whether it's worth carrying an umbrella [10].

2. *Different types of data and how they require different types of analysis.* How can we tell whether data is "normal" and if it is not, should we use a non-parametric test, transform the data, or something else? Why are length of stay, costs, and other such variables considered "count data," and how should count data be handled? What are the causes and consequences of incomplete data, and how should we address the missing data in the analysis?

3. *Specific research scenarios.* Any research is driven by questions – what are the risks for a complication, for example, and how can we estimate or constrain them? What are examples of useful research questions? How do research questions at the clinical level translate to practical issues

at the analysis level? Is it possible to do too many tests, and how do we ensure that results are relevant to patients outside our study? How do we distinguish the clinical difference from statistical difference?

4. *Presenting results.* Lastly, we will review good practices for interpreting and presenting results so your findings come across quickly and clearly.

Arguably, a statistical association can be described in one of three ways:

1. *Yes, the association is large enough to influence decision-making.* This possibility may include the case where the p-value is not significant or the case if the confidence interval (CI) includes a range of values that would be grounds for action if statistically significant. In the worst case, we design and carry out a more appropriate study. "More appropriate" may mean more subjects to improve the statistical power but may also mean a more careful selection of patients or the measurement of data that allows a clearer assessment of treatment mechanisms and outcomes.

2. *The association is small enough to be considered negligible.* This is separate from the p-value; a finding can be statistically significant but very small such as an increase in life expectancy of less than a day. Although this may not be as desirable as a finding that leads to improved patient care, clinical efficiency should be improved by reducing the number of things to be considered. Additionally, identifying and eliminating unnecessary tests or procedures may protect the patient from potential adverse events. However, making this statement assumes that we can estimate the factor with enough precision that we can say even its most extreme values are too small to worry about; otherwise we have to consider.

3. *We can't tell with the immediately available data.* This is the least desirable case, but the results do not necessarily leave the patient, clinician, or care organization worse off. We may have to design a new study or drop the project for now, since the study design may not allow a meaningful answer to our question or the sample size may be too small. As we will discuss, saying "we don't know" is less likely to do harm than claiming a meaningful finding and being in error. On the other hand, we have to distinguish between not being able to support an association and being able to prove that there is no association; this is succinctly phrased as "absence of evidence is not evidence of absence" [11].

We would also add caution here that even in a significant study where the confidence interval includes effects large enough to have a clinical impact, if the confidence interval is wide enough (say, in a small study) that the confidence interval also includes negligible effects, we may not be able to properly distinguish between cases 1 and 2 – and so wind up with case 3, we can't tell!

CHAPTER 2

Interpreting Probability: Medical School Axioms of Probability

"PROBABILITY," LIKE "HEALTH," IS a word that everyone uses intuitively, without thinking of the precise definition. However, anyone planning a research study has had to deal with exact definitions of diagnoses and/or treatments. In this chapter, we discuss various ways of defining probability and relate them to clinical expectations. Telling a patient "this is your most probable outcome" may be misleading if the patient and the surgeon use different definitions of probability.

Imagine that you have a patient who needs to undergo a procedure with a 4% risk of complication. Does that mean that if you could somehow perform 100 identical operations on the same patient, you would expect four to result in complications? What about performing the same operation on each of 100 identical patients? How does that 4% risk resolve into contributions from

11

patient susceptibility, errors during the surgical procedure, and simple random chance, such as whether a blood clot will form? For our artificial scenarios, the patient's susceptibility should be fixed. Now let's take this example one step further – 100 identical patients are all getting the same operation, but each one from a different surgeon. Differences between surgeons now have to be accounted for. Finally, let's repeat these 100-surgery trials 1,000 times – not 1,000 surgeries but each of these 100-surgery sets repeated 1,000 times, with the same combination of the patient, operation, and surgery in each cycle. Will the same four patients or the same four surgeons have a complication with each iteration?

These what-if's illustrate how murky the mathematical idea of probability can be. Abelson [2] points out that the generation of random data is something different from the random sampling of a fixed population, even though we may not be able to distinguish the two in the data we see. You might view probability in the sense of the ancient Greek line that you can never step in the same river twice. The water may flow at a constant rate along a fixed path, but it's not the same water (temperature, microorganisms, etc.) from moment to moment. The flow is the probability, and the moment you step into it is the instance of data collection.

Consider a potential data set for surgeries. The data includes the patient getting the operation and the surgeon(s) performing the operation and the outcomes of the operation: blood loss, what complications occurred, and so on. We can describe the patients by observable variables such as age, ethnicity, gender, blood type, height, weight, ethnicity, comorbidities, lab tests, or prior surgeries. We could similarly describe the surgeons by their years of experience, specific training, or the number of surgeries done. The surgery itself can be captured as time on the table, surgical approach, and type of anesthesia used. (None of these sample lists are comprehensive – it is often possible to record more variables than patients, which is a problem in itself we will consider in Chapter 11.) We expect that some patients will be at greater risk than others, but not that any given patient is doomed to a complication. We also expect that some minimum risk is unavoidable. One possible goal of a statistical analysis is to determine whether a specific factor affects patient outcomes. Another possible goal is to estimate the typical outcome for patients. But are these two goals the same thing, and are they the only options? We expect that some surgeons may perform better than others, everything else being equal; perhaps we are comparing surgeons who prefer one method and those who prefer another.

When grappling with large questions, a useful approach is to find simple scenarios that approximate the more complicated situations. For example, take a roulette wheel. You don"t have to visit Las Vegas to know what a roulette wheel is. The little ball drops into the spinning wheel and eventually winds up in a little slot. What the ball does on one spin is not related to what it will do on another spin. The ball's behavior can be readily described in terms of frequencies. Assuming these gambling games are honest, the frequencies will be the same on any visit to any casino. This is one simple way to imagine probability. Decks of cards and rolls of dice have also been seen as examples in statistical texts.

At this point, we should acknowledge that we are using what is known as a *frequentist* view of probability. Probability is defined by the frequency of observing certain events. That event might be whether a complication occurs or doesn't occur, or it might be whether a lab value is within a certain range. This "frequentist" view is not the only way of viewing probability but it is the method most common in the medical literature as of this writing. The leading contender is the *Bayesian* view, which sees probability as the strength of belief in an outcome happening, to be updated by accumulated evidence and by a useful tool called Bayes' theorem, from which Bayesian statistics gets its name. Bayes' theorem has applications in the frequentist framework, for example, in defining the relationship between sensitivity and the positive predictive value, which we will discuss in more detail in Chapter 8.

We also assume here that the quantity of interest can be chopped into arbitrarily small pieces. Time, for example, can be divided into years, days, minutes, seconds, nanoseconds, and so on. Money, on the other hand, has certain fixed minimum units – in America, what are fractions of a cent? – but when a large number of values are possible for a single variable, it can be treated as a continuous number. But the question "how many days a week are you physically active?" can be answered only with values 0 through 7. We will discuss how to handle these special cases of count data in Chapter 12.

Getting away from gambling examples, let's go to a physical location that you're familiar with – an office, a classroom, or a restaurant (which, arguably, may still be in or near Las Vegas) – and find the average age of the people there. Then, repeat the same measurement again exactly one week later in the same environment. Would you get the same number? Even if the same people are expected to be there on a regular schedule, for example, those enrolled in a class or working in an office, not everyone will be there every day. Some will be on vacation or out sick during either of the two weeks used for measurement. No one is expected to randomly get older or younger, although each person has a 1-in-52 chance of having had a birthday in the intervening week. Thus, even though age is a fixed quantity, the average age of the group is a random variable based on the chance of being present. You would expect similar results using height, although that might show some variation based on shoes worn that day. Weight is expected to be a variable, as it is known to vary day to day for the same person.

In statistics, variations that we can anticipate but which we cannot explicitly account for are usually lumped together into one "random error." This error is usually assumed to follow a well-known bell-shaped distribution that is alternatively called the Gaussian or normal distribution (Figure 2.1A). The Gaussian distribution is very convenient. It can be completely defined by two parameters, the mean and the standard deviation (SD),

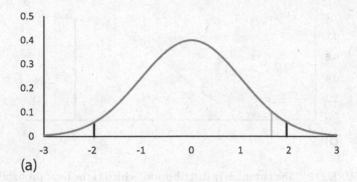
(a)

FIGURE 2.1A The Gaussian probability distribution from three different perspectives. A is the bell-shaped probability density function, which shows the probability of a variable with mean 0 and SD 1 having a particular value. The black bars indicate the breakpoints of ±1.96, where the total probability of being outside those lines (less than −1.96 or greater than 1.96) is 5%. The gray bar indicates the breakpoint of 1.64, and the total probability of being greater than 1.64 is 5%. (This is the basis of the two-tailed versus one-tailed test.)

which you've met in statistics classes and which we will consider in Chapter 3. In Figure 2.1A, the mean is 0 and the SD is 1.

Assuming a defined distribution, Gaussian or not, allows researchers to make statements about the precision of the estimate and how likely the observations were to arise from random chance. Statistical tools such as t-tests and regressions base their results on the assumption that the variation not accounted for by group membership or predictor variables will follow a Gaussian distribution. The basis of this assumption is an important principle of probability, the *central limit theorem*, which states that the sum of multiple random variables can follow a Gaussian distribution even if the original variables are not themselves Gaussian. The mean, of course, is the sum of measurements divided by the number of measurements.

Any probability distribution can also be redefined as a *cumulative distribution function*, which describes the probability that the observed value will be above or below a certain amount. The

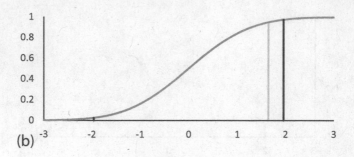

(b)

FIGURE 2.1B The cumulative distribution, which is the total probability of the variable having a value at or below some threshold. It is the summation of all points in 2.1A to the left of a particular value; note the inflection at 0 (the peak in 2.1A). The black and gray bars from 2.1A are drawn for the context. The cumulative distribution at −1.96 is 2.5%, the cumulative distribution at +1.96 is 97.5%, and that at 1.64 is 95%. In a statistical test, the p-value is the probability of the test statistic being at or above some threshold value.

cumulative distribution function for the Gaussian in Figure 2.1A is shown in Figure 2.1B. Half of the values are above the mean of 0, and half are below the mean, so the cumulative probability at the mean is 50%.

Any mathematical function can be a probability distribution if it follows two rules: (1) it can never be less than zero; otherwise, you'd have a negative probability of an event; and 2) the sum of all its possible values is 100%, the probability that at least one of the values in the distribution will be observed. For example, Figure 2.1C shows a lognormal distribution, which is a skewed distribution (not symmetric) and also one in which no values can be at or below zero.

If you want to get the probability of a value being between two boundaries A and B, where A is less than B, then you subtract the probability of the value being greater than B from the (larger) probability of the value being greater than the smaller value A. Thus, a 95% confidence interval is defined by the extremes where there is a 2.5% probability of being at or below

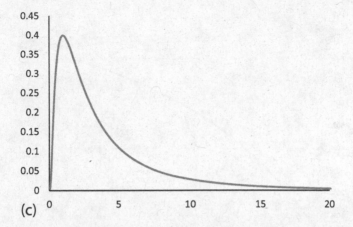

FIGURE 2.1C The lognormal distribution is the same function as 2.1A, but the axis is transformed by the exponential function. So the X-axis in 2.1C is the exponential of the X-axis in 2.A, or alternatively the X-axis in 2.1A is the natural logarithm of the X-axis in 2.1C.

the lower bound and a 2.5% probability of being at or above the higher bound: 100% − 2.5% − 2.5% = 95%. For the convenient Gaussian distribution, the 95% CI can be defined by the estimate ± 1.96 times the standard error (SE), which is the SD divided by the square root of the sample size. Reflecting this, Figures 2.1A and 2.1B show the locations of the 2.5% and 97.5% bounds (black vertical lines, at ±1.96) in the cumulative function. They also show the location of the 95% bound (1.64), where the total probability above that bound is 5%. These boundaries are familiar conventions in statistical tests, as discussed in Chapters 4 and 5.

Let's return to the medical school adages we mentioned earlier from the perspective of probability:

HORSES BEFORE ZEBRAS

A high-probability event is, by definition, more likely than a low-probability event. However, if the probability is greater than zero, then the expectation is that a low-probability event will inevitably

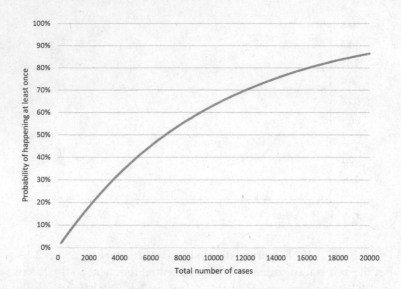

FIGURE 2.2   The increasing probability of a rare event being observed at least once as the total number of cases increases. This is implemented as an Excel sheet so the baseline values can be tweaked. In this example, the baseline probability is 0.01%.

be seen. If the probability of an event is P, then the probability of not seeing it is $(1 - P)$ on a single case, and the probability of not seeing it in N cases is $(1 - P)^N$. This is shown visually in Figure 2.2, which is also implemented as an Excel example – you can change both P and N. If a specific condition will only be seen in 1/10,000 patients, then a surgeon who sees 20,000 patients over a period will expect to see two patients with that condition. However, that does not mean every surgeon will see 2/20,000 of a specific condition; there is a $(1 - 1/10,000)^{20,000} = 13.5\%$ chance that a surgeon seeing 20,000 patients will never see any with that condition (this touches on why count data needs to be handled specially). Similarly, if the surgery has a 4% complication rate, and we predict as a general rule that "the patient will not have a complication," we will be right 96% of the time, but is that sufficient? A better strategy would be to assume horses first, but be prepared for zebras. Simple explanations are good but not too simple, which brings us to the next section.

THE SIMPLEST EXPLANATION IS MOST LIKELY

Let's assume that the more complicated an explanation is, the more events it depends on. For example, let's consider a postoperative infection. First, the bacteria must be present. Then it has to get into the patient's system. Then it has to elude the body's defenses and grow. What is the likelihood of the infection being polymicrobial (more than one organism)? More than one organism must have the opportunity to get into the system, and each of them has to thrive. If these are independent events, where the occurrence of one event has no effect on the chance of another happening, then the total probability of the event is the product $P1 * P2$, up to Pn, where n is the total number of necessary events for the complicated explanation, and Pj is the probability of the jth event in the chain and j is between 1 and n. All probabilities are bounded between 0 and 1, so the probability of every event occurring will be less than the probability of any single event in the set. Polymicrobial infections are uncommon, but they can happen. Proverbs are generalizations, so they have exceptions.

THE PATIENT CAN HAVE AS MANY DISEASES AS THEY PLEASE

If we are dealing with independent events, the probability of multiple events occurring is the product of their individual probabilities – so the probability of multiple diseases would be the product of the chances of having each disease, and it doesn't matter which disease was acquired first. However, it may not be realistic to assume that patient comorbidities are independent. If the patient is already suffering from one condition, then weakened defenses or the relative lack of exercise may increase vulnerability to acquire or suffer others. In any event, the only thing preventing a patient from acquiring conditions indefinitely is mortality.

THERE ARE MORE DIFFERENCES BETWEEN BAD MEDICINE AND GOOD MEDICINE; THAN THERE IS BETWEEN GOOD MEDICINE AND NO MEDICINE

The expected *net* benefit of good medicine can be described, paralleling the definition of expected value, as the probability of the benefit being realized multiplied by the magnitude of the potential benefit from treatment, minus the risk of side-effects multiplied by the magnitude of the harm from the side-effects. In an equation, Net = P(Benefit) * (Benefit from Treatment) – P(Risk) * (Harm from Side-Effects). If the treatment has no potential benefit, so at least one of P(Benefit) or (Benefit from Treatment) is zero, the treatment may still have side-effects or complications, while a patient who does not get the treatment will not get any additional harm.

Obviously, a life without risk is impossible, and decisions have to balance risks and benefits. Avoiding surgery for fear of complications, plunging ahead into surgery without considering the risks, and buying lottery tickets as an investment are all variations of the same mistake: being guided by the magnitude of the potential outcome and not by its probability. Therefore, it is important that clinical studies be carefully planned, analyzed, and reviewed prior to publication: decisions can be hurt by misinformation.

CHAPTER 3

Statistics, the Law of Large Numbers, and the Confidence Interval

A STATISTIC, SINGULAR, IS A calculated value which will estimate some property of a collection of numbers. The mean, for example, estimates the typical value for a single variable, and the standard deviation (SD) estimates how far off you might be if you assume the mean value in the absence of an actual measurement. These estimates are subject to how much spread is already in the data. If you're measuring age from a homogeneous population – say, students in a classroom – you would see less variation than, for example, among people in a supermarket. (We're setting aside the question of extreme values, also known as outliers, for the moment.)

Say we have two classrooms in the same school, both the same grade with a similar distribution of males and females, and we compare average heights. Do we expect the two averages to be equal? Realistically, no, because we would expect some variation between groups. Even for a given classroom, some students may be out on any given day and you might have a difference between measurements for the same classroom on different days. However, in the language of statistics, both groups would have the same expected value (average height) and the variation between them would be a separate quantity. If we estimated the average height, we would expect the averages from each group would be a bit different from the true average because of random variation. This is why estimates come with confidence intervals (CIs) or margins of error.

A possible consequence of even small errors in estimation can be seen in Figure 3.1. Let's assume that we're interested in classifying a patient as abnormal if some lab value is more than 2 SD below the mean. That's about 2.5% of patients. The offset between the Gaussian curves, representing 15% of an SD difference between estimation and reality, is just large enough to detect by the eye, as is the corresponding offset between the cumulative functions. However, if you look at the ratio between curves, the difference is about 40%: 3.5%, not 2.5%, of patients may show up based on the threshold.

All statistical estimates are subject to the *law of large numbers*, which states that as the number of observations increases, the margin for error in estimates will improve. The concept here can be shown with a simple example: assume we've flipped a coin and had an unusual streak of ten heads. Then, assume we continue flipping the coin N number of times. For an ideal coin, we expect 50% of flips will be heads, so the observed probability of heads will be $(10 + N/2)/N$, or $\frac{1}{2} + 10/N$. As N increases to infinity, the $10/N$ term drops toward zero and the observed probability approaches $\frac{1}{2}$. You can try this for yourself with different values of N or set it up in Excel (Figure 3.2). You'll notice that at a certain point, even large increases in N do not return any meaningful improvement in the estimate.

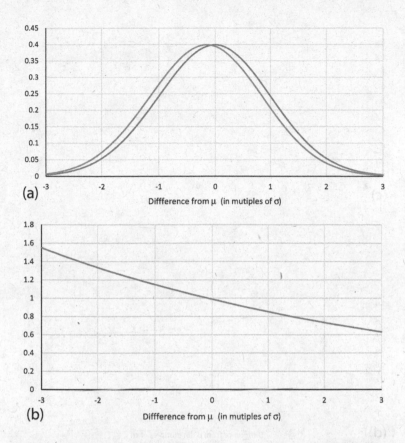

(a) Diffference from μ (in mutiples of σ)

(b) Diffference from μ (in mutiples of σ)

FIGURE 3.1 A: The normal distribution as seen in 2.1A but with a slight shift 0.15 in the mean (implemented in Excel so you can examine the impact). This shift might be a real thing (differences between two populations) or a consequence of the estimation error. B: The ratio between values observed due to the shift. C: Cumulative normal distribution, the same shift. Also implemented in Excel. The effect of the offset is more visible in the middle (near 0). D: Relative effect on the cumulative normal distribution, as the ratio of the two curves. The relative effect of the offset is greatest at smaller values, decreasing as the difference from the mean increases.

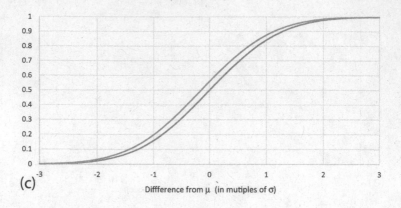

(c)

Diffference from μ (in mutiples of σ)

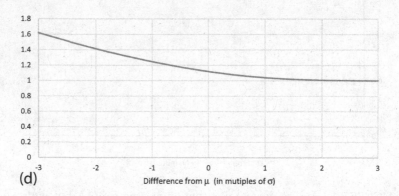

(d)

Diffference from μ (in mutiples of σ)

FIGURE 3.1 (Continued)

The law of large numbers is often misunderstood as the "law of averages," also known as the gambler's fallacy, which is the assumption that an outcome that has not happened recently has a higher probability of happening. As shown above, the final estimate only depends on the number of outcomes, not on the history or any connection between subsequent events. If you flip a coin three times and get three heads, you are not "due" a fourth. In the short term, to quote Robert Abelson, the chance is lumpy [2]. It can be frightening to realize that a streak – say, a series of

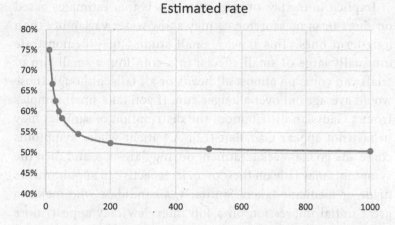

FIGURE 3.2 Statistical estimates may appear extreme for small samples but per the law of large numbers will approach the true estimate as the sample size increases. In this example (also implemented in Excel) there has been a run of 10/10 "positives" for a binary variable with a true value of 50%. The curve shows how the estimate will be expected to approach the true value with additional samples, assuming the samples have a mean positive rate of the true value.

operations that turn out very well or all have complications – may depend on a chance at least as much as the performance of the clinician. (This assumes, of course, that nothing else is varying over time or between clinicians. Assessing and controlling for that is considered in Chapter 11.)

If we're within 0.1% of the true value, what do we gain by getting to within 0.01% or 0.001%, and how big does N have to be to get to that range of precision? The margin of error decreases with the square root of N; if we have four times the number of samples, the uncertainty is cut in half. If we have a dataset with hundreds of patients and then another handful become available, we do not expect our statistical estimates to change much, unless something very unusual has happened. If you've ever said to a statistician "good news, we found another few patients!" and got a jaundiced look, now you know why.

Implicit in the law of large numbers is that estimates based on short-term measurements may show wider variability than long-term ones. This is why small studies may demonstrate unusually large or small effects; in a coin flip, a small run of trials can come up almost all heads or all tails, although these would average out over a longer run. If you take small samples from a Gaussian distribution, the distribution of samples may in fact not appear Gaussian [12]. A patient whose symptoms come and go may seek treatment during flare-ups, and then the symptoms may fade on their own, irrespective of appointments made or medicine taken. Similarly, a candidate who makes a great initial impression on a job interview may appear more mediocre when they start. A bad day will be followed by a better one, a good day by a worse one. Small hospitals may seem to have extremes, good and bad, of figures of merit such as the complication rate. There is no law of averages, just a phenomenon that statisticians call *regression to the mean* – extremes are followed by less extreme values.

Yes, the phenomenon of regression to the mean is associated with the method of regression. In a straight-line regression of Y on X, $Y = A^*X + B + e$, where e is the random error term and A and B are the regression intercept and slope, respectively. Let's describe the variability of X with the standard deviation S_x. The expected variability of Y is A^*S_x, but the observed variability of Y is $A^*S_x + e$. So tall parents might have children who were taller than average but are not expected to be as tall as or taller than their parents, and the distribution of qualities across the human race remains fairly constant across time. There is also a *regression fallacy* where, in individual cases, the random variation is confused with the effect of intervention – such as the perceived response of a patient to treatment or a student to reward or punishment. The individual patient or student might have shown improvement over the course of time. Valid inferences have to be drawn on the effect of the intervention across the population, all things being equal (for how to get there, see Chapter 11).

The variability in an estimate of the mean can be described by the standard error, which is the SD divided by the square root of the sample size. The 95% CI is defined by the mean ± 1.96 × the standard error, the 1.96 coming from the mathematics of the Gaussian distribution. The standard deviation is itself an estimate. The t-distribution, which is the basis of Student's t-test, takes that into account, and for a large enough sample size (>30 or so), the Gaussian and the t-distribution overlap. The estimated mean plus or minus 1.96 times the SD should capture 95% of the possible values in the population, with 2.5% below the lower bound (mean − 1.96 SD) and 2.5% above the upper bound (mean + 1.96 SD). Thus, the 95% CI is defined by the mean ± 1.96 × the standard error (SD/sqrt(N)), and the assumption is that we can be 95% sure the mean is within this range. That is, if we repeated the same sampling and calculation many times, getting a new CI each time, 95% of the CIs would contain the true mean.

This holds whether you are looking at a continuous value (e.g. age or body mass index [BMI]) or a categorical outcome (e.g. complication – yes or no). If you replace no with 0 and yes with 1, then the average is the estimated proportion of patients with the outcome subject to the variation error. A statistician once accidentally provoked an argument with the maintainer of a data set who had dutifully recorded every instance of a complication. The statistician gratefully stated that we have a good estimate of the complication rate, to which the maintainer grumbled that it wasn't an estimate; it was the actual rate. The statistical point was that the observed rate and the underlying probability were not the same things. Otherwise, every time you flipped a coin 2N times, you would always get N heads.

The CI represents a range of the plausible values of the mean, and a narrower CI (either from smaller SD or larger N) indicates a smaller margin for error. A CI can be calculated for any statistic, not just the mean. The calculation can be based on the mathematics of the assumed probability distribution or on a technique called "bootstrapping," where a given sample is repeatedly resampled – with some subjects dropped and others included more than once – to create a range of plausible possible values.

CHAPTER 4

The Basics of Statistical Tests

CARE AND FEEDING OF p-VALUES

A statistic does not just have to summarize a single variable. A statistical test summarizes the association between measurements of interest (such as treatment and outcome) in a single number called a test statistic. This test statistic is compared against a known distribution, which might not be Gaussian, and the *p-value* estimates that probability for which a value of at least that observed test statistic would have happened, *if* it is true that the measurements of interest are in fact *not* related. This assumption is called the *null hypothesis* since it can be generally stated as the assumption that the expected difference between the two groups is zero (that is, null). Expressed another way, if two groups have the same distribution, then the null hypothesis is that the expected measurement from one is the same as the expected measurement from another. (If the two groups do not have the same distribution – perhaps one has a wider variance or is more skewed – then there's something going on you should investigate.) There is also a variation called a *sharp* null hypothesis, which assumes for every individual in a group, the expected effect of a treatment is zero; this is different from the expectation that some patients may get better and some worse, so the expected average effect is zero.

It's been argued that the null hypothesis will almost never be true because each group is subject to random variation and so the difference between identically distributed groups may never be exactly zero. For example, if we take the average heights of two first-grade classes in the same school, we will not get the exact same number, but the difference between average heights will be negligibly small compared to the variation within classes. To repeat: the null hypothesis declares that the expected values are the same, not the observed values. You could find an inch of difference between the two means but be unable to reject the null hypothesis if the margin of error is plus or minus an inch and a half. Even if you reject the null hypothesis, the observed difference between groups is likely to be a mix of a systematic difference and the chance variation. You can view a statistical test as trying to assess which potential explanation of the observed data is the least incompatible with the evidence.

A statistical model such as a t-test or regression will try to estimate both the systematic difference and the random variation. Usually these calculations assume that the random variation follows a Gaussian distribution. This assumption is violated not only if the difference does not follow a Gaussian distribution but also if there are covariates affecting the outcomes which are not accounted for in the statistical model. Chapter 11 discusses how to account for the covariates, while Chapter 12 discusses options if the error component is not Gaussian. To understand why the Gaussian assumption is important, consider the common situation where the measurement error increases with the average measurement; for example, if you plot the length of stay versus cost, you may see that there is more scatter around the larger values of either. If the standard deviation is constant, then a difference of X dollars or days would be the same number of standard deviations wherever you started. However, if the standard deviation varies, then X would be a smaller change where the standard deviation was larger. One reason to transform data is to stabilize the variance so that the same statistical properties hold over the range of the data.

The familiar routine of "null hypothesis significance testing" (which is a name given to it in the literature, often by papers critiquing the approach) is actually a compromise between two historical approaches to statistical tests developed in the 1920s and 1930s, and the combination is still considered controversial in the statistical community. On the one hand, Ronald Fisher saw a statistical test as a way to estimate how strongly accumulated evidence weighed against the null hypothesis. Jerzy Neyman and Egon Pearson developed a more rigorous mathematical approach aimed at comparing two hypotheses, including details such as Type I and Type II error, the size of an effect, and the calculation of a sample size. A detailed review of differences between Fisher, Neyman-Pearson, and the hybrid approach [13] summarizes the hybrid testing approach you are probably familiar with, as the following "Neyman-Pearson procedurally but Fisher philosophically." That review and a more mathematical one [14] point out that the Fisher and Neyman-Pearson perspectives can often converge to the same result, but they do exhibit philosophical differences. The reviews agree that the solution is to think about the problem rather than apply an automatic procedure.

You may have heard something of the debate over p-values. We will get into further detail later in this book, but our position is that the p-value has real but limited utility in assessing whether a visible change is promising. A significant p-value by itself may have no real meaning to the clinician or patient. For example, two weight-loss plans may have p-values of 0.001 and 0.10, the first being significant and the second, not. But suppose the average weight loss of the first plan was 6 ounces, and that of the second plan was 40 pounds.

The p-value should also *never* be used as a goal – that is, do not keep tinkering with the analyses until you get a low p-value. This is an example of what in economics is called Goodhart's Law: when a measure becomes a target, it ceases to be a measure. You might as well shoot an arrow into a wall and then draw a bull's-eye around the arrow.

The p-value tells us how likely it is that we observed the differences we did, *if* it were true that random variation is the only explanation. (This is one reason not to use the p-value as a target – if you've kept sifting through analyses until you get an acceptable p-value, the act of searching takes the probability out of the p-value.) The lower the p-value, the less credible the null hypothesis. But a high p-value cannot be seen as proof that the null hypothesis is true, only that the data is insufficient to reject it. There is an additional assumption: the statistical test was appropriate for the problem at hand. You may remember from statistics class that Type I error is rejecting the null hypothesis when it is actually true, and Type II error is not rejecting the null hypothesis when it is in fact false. It may be said that Type III error may have had the wrong null hypothesis in the first place – the study began with the wrong research question.

There is an alternative approach to p-values we will discuss here to help clarify how they represent the probability of results arising from random chances given the null hypothesis being true. The permutation test can be computationally expensive and is only useful in simple study designs, but the underlying concept is straightforward. For many iterations, repeat the statistical test after scrambling the order of the outcome, so you are performing repeated tests based on the assumption that the outcome was generated purely randomly. The p-value in this context is the rate at which the randomized iterations outscore the original test. For example, consider comparing the means between two groups. In the permutation test, use the difference between groups as the test statistic. If there is a systematic difference between groups, then few, if any, of the randomized datasets should show a larger difference than the original data and the permutation p-value will be low. If no such systematic difference exists, then the p-value would be much higher. If we are only interested in changes in one direction, say showing that group B minus group A is greater than 0, then we would ask how often the permuted difference in means (which may be positive or negative) is greater than that in the original data. If we want a two-sided test, where we want to show that A and B are different, then we would use the absolute value of the differences but still ask how often the permuted difference is larger in magnitude than the original difference.

The American Statistical Association has issued a statement [15] that summarizes what information a p-value can and cannot provide. This statement is recommended for reading. We would not dismiss the p-value as useless but would point out it is merely one piece of information. A low p-value suggests that the finding shows a consistent difference between groups relative to the inherent uncertainty in the measurements. A p-value above 0.05 but still around 0.15 or so may suggest that the study would have returned the desired p-value with larger sample size. This is different from adding more patients and re-running, which is equivalent to using the p-value as a target and declaring the study finished when a significant p-value has been reached. A high p-value, by itself, cannot distinguish between not having enough data and the lack of an effect; as the saying goes, "absence of evidence is not evidence of absence" [11].

THE PERILS OF PRODUCTIVITY

The familiar convention that a p-value less than 0.05 is "significant" is based on the idea that the probability of rejecting the null hypothesis, given that the null hypothesis is actually true, should be 5% or less. But that 5% is not trivial. Imagine that 20 different researchers all get the same idea for a research project, and the null hypothesis is true, which of course may not be known for certain beforehand or after. If the probability of a "significant" test result is 5%, given that the null hypothesis is true, then we can reasonably expect that of the 20 researchers; one of them will find a statistically significant p-value less than 0.05 through chance alone, and the lucky (?) author will write up the results for publication, while the other 19 will move on to other projects. Conversely, an author may find that an expected relationship is not present in the analyzed data and therefore submit the paper believing it's a novel finding and not just a random fluke. This can make productivity counter-productive.

The "Spurious Correlations" website at https://www.tylervig en.com/spurious-correlations shows how, if you compare and contrast enough variables, any two will appear to covary even though there is no logical connection between them (for example, accidental drownings correlating with the film roles of Nicholas Cage). This is one reason to be cautious using large administrative databases. An exploration of 53 drug-outcome pairs across 10 observational databases [16] showed that there could be a considerable divergence in statistical findings, with 11/53 cohort comparisons showing both statistically significant increases and decreases in risk.

The matter is approached with more mathematical rigor in a paper available freely online called "Why Most Published Research Findings Are False," by John Ioannidis [17], whose provocative title gives an idea of how much debate has gone on since Ronald Fisher and Jerzy Neyman began arguing about hypothesis testing in the 1930s. Dr. Ionnadis has also written a follow-up paper called "How to Make More Published Research True" from which one recommendation is to spread the awareness of more appropriate statistical methods [18]. Andrew Gelman [19] describes how a researcher may select the analysis methods based on the observations of the data, like Sherlock Holmes following clues, but wind up biasing results based on selecting certain analysis methods as opposed to other equally appropriate methods. Even though the researchers are conscientious and sincere, the net effect is to bias the results in favor of false positives even though no deliberate attempt to mislead the investigation was intended.

SAMPLE SIZE VERSUS p-VALUES

The law of large numbers can play a role here. Keep in mind that the p-value is calculated based on three factors, two of which are estimates: the estimated difference between groups and the SD within groups. The third factor is the sample size. The p-value becomes smaller as the difference between groups or the sample size increases and becomes larger as the variation increases. As you increase the sample size, the estimated mean and SD approach their true values and stay there, so the p-value will decrease steadily and even negligible associations will become statistically significant with high enough N. For smaller studies, the law of large numbers would indicate a wider variation in the estimates of both means and SDs, so both the effect size and its p-value can be distorted [20]. This wide variation can lead to false positives in the literature: if several researchers independently work on the same research question with their own small data sets, only one of them may get what seems to be a meaningful finding and that study will be submitted for publication while the others get dropped.

There's another element of sample size that does not seem to be considered in practice. Since the margin for error per group is controlled by the sample size within each group, per the law of large numbers, the overall uncertainty is dominated by the size of the smallest group. The effective sample size per group is not the total number of patients divided by the total number of groups, but (brace yourselves) the reciprocal of the mean of the reciprocals of patients per group. So if there were 10 in one group and 30 in another, the effective sample size per group would *not* be $40/2 = 20$ but would be $1/(0.5 * (1/10+1/15)) = 15$! Even though you have 40 patients, the imbalance means you have the same statistical power as if you had 30 patients in a balanced study of 15 each. The difference of 20 patients between groups effectively only gains you another 10 because of the imbalance. In a more abstract way, assume you have N patients in one group and $c \times N$ (where c doesn't have to be an integer) in the other. Then, the effective

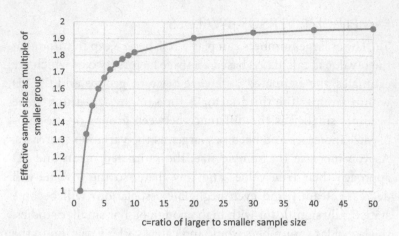

FIGURE 4.1 As you combine two populations of different sample sizes, the effective sample size for your statistical test will be weighted toward the smaller sample size. Beyond a rate of 5:1, there are clear diminishing returns.

sample size per group is $2c/(c + 1)$ times N. If c is 1, then $2c/(c+1) = 1.0$. As c goes up to infinity, you can't do better than 2N for an effective sample size. The situation is plotted in Figure 4.1. For c of 3, you have 1.5N per group; for c of 5, you have 1.67N per group. If you're doing a study where data acquisition may be labor-intensive, consider where the point of diminishing returns may be. Also, bear in mind that if your goal is to estimate probabilities, then you may require the actual ratios of cases and controls.

ALWAYS INCLUDE THE CONFIDENCE INTERVAL

A useful relative of the p-value is the confidence interval (CI, Figure 4.2), which can describe the degree of uncertainty in estimates and the size of the effect [21]. Figure 4.2 does not show concrete numbers because the line of "no change" might be a value of 0 if we were looking at net differences between quantities such as the length of stay or cost, but it might be 1 if we were talking about odds ratios or hazard ratios. A CI can be drawn for any parameter – net difference, odds ratio, hazard ratio, etc.

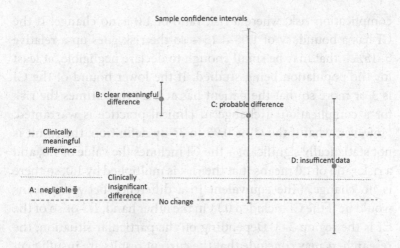

FIGURE 4.2 Hypothetical confidence intervals in different scenarios. In A, the effect is statistically distinct from 0 but is not clinically meaningful. In B, the effect is both clinically and statistically significant. In C, the effect is not statistically significant, but this may be a consequence of insufficient statistical power; consider a new study with more data or patients likelier to show a larger response. In D, the data doesn't allow for any clear statement to be made.

Note that frequentist statistics' "competitor" Bayesian statistics does not have p-values at all but does use a variation of CI. As we would expect from the law of large numbers, higher sample sizes result in a narrower CI as well as lower p-values, reflecting better estimates up to the point where the improvement in precision becomes vanishingly small. Knowing either CI or p-value, you can calculate the other [22, 23].

The CI is arguably more useful than a p-value because it describes not only what the estimated difference is between groups but also how much precision is in that estimate. The exact interpretation of the CI depends not only on the statistical tools used to derive it but also on the clinician being able to answer at least one of two questions: what difference between groups is too small to care about, and what difference between groups is large enough to justify the action? Let's say we're looking at the complication risk, where a risk ratio of 1.0 is no change. If the CI has a boundary of 1.05–1.15 – so the risk goes up a relative 5–15% – that may be small enough to declare negligible, at least for the population being studied. If the lower bound of the CI is 3 or more so that the patient has at least three times the risk for a complication, a change in clinical practice is warranted. However, what if the CI is 0.95 to 3? By definition, the result is not statistically significant – the CI includes the value of 1.0, and a risk ratio of 1.0 means that the risk is multiplied by 1.0, so there is no change. (The equivalent in a difference between means would be if the CI included 0.) On the other hand, 1/3 or so of the CI is the region 2–3. Depending on the particular situation, the researchers may conclude that the current results are insufficient to make a definitive statement or perhaps that the possibility of a twofold or more increase in the risk is enough to justify action.

Also note that if two CIs overlap – say, for outcome scores in two surgical groups – it does not necessarily mean that there is no statistically distinct difference between them. To establish that, you want the confidence interval for the difference itself.

CHAPTER 5

How Much Data Is Enough?

IF INCREASING THE AMOUNT of data improves the precision of an estimate, then it would follow that there is some minimum amount of data required to make a statistical case. So how much data is enough? This has to be considered in any prospective study, where you have to plan and justify recruitment numbers. If you are working from an administrative database, then the amount of data is fixed and is probably large unless you are looking at rare conditions present in only a small fraction of patients.

The ability to detect an effect is what statisticians call power. If the study does not have enough statistical power to test a specific hypothesis, then an analysis may not be useful to make statements about whether the factor of interest has the hypothesized effect. A study with low statistical power is also not likely to provide estimates with useful precision. Whether you are trying to estimate the effect of a treatment, estimate the prognosis of a patient of a particular age, or just get some insight into the relationships between two physiological measurements, the math is the same.

Sample size analyses try to estimate how many subjects are needed for adequate statistical power. These analyses are often based on a mathematical quantity called *effect size*. The exact definition varies between tests, but for a t-test, it's simply the difference between means divided by the SD of the continuous outcome variable. (This is similar to but not the same as the test statistic for the t-test, which is the mean divided by the standard error.) Overall, an effect size is dimensionless – for example, mean and SD both have the same units, so mean/SD is dimensionless (as is mean/SE). Smaller effect sizes require larger sample sizes to demonstrate statistically significant differences, and the null hypothesis is an effect size of 0. Ideally, sample size planning for a prospective study should explicitly assess how much variation is in the data and how much difference between groups is expected or meaningful. These might be determined by reviewing the literature for similar studies where the means and SDs have been published, by reviewing data on hand in an administrative database to see how measurements are distributed, or by conducting a small pilot study.

A statistician named Jacob Cohen suggested that in the absence of relevant data, each test could use a pre-defined "small," "medium," or "large" effect size [24, 25]. This is controversial because it is a cookbook approach that does not consider the actual data; it can be a useful way to jump-start a study, but the researcher should consider whether plausible and meaningful measurable effects are consistent with Cohen's suggested effect sizes. There is also a surprising argument for the use of Cohen's "medium" effect size of 0.5 for (mean difference)/SD – in a review of patient-reported outcomes [26], it was found that the minimally important difference divided by the standard deviation per test tended to be about 0.495 (with an SD of 0.15 across tests); the authors suggested an explanation might be that half a standard deviation was the bottom limit of human discrimination. Cohen stated [24] he selected 0.5 as a "medium" effect size because it was "likely to be visible to the naked eye of a careful observer."

The classic ways of estimating sample size for statistical tests are covered in detail in statistical books and conveniently implemented at the site www.sealedenvelope.com or in the free G*Power 3 program available at http://gpower.hhu.de. Remember, similar to the 5% Type I error rate, the Type II error rate of 20% (80% power) is a convention, not a law. There are situations where you may want to loosen or tighten either of them. Looser constraints allow for smaller sample sizes. However, please remember our warnings not to get too wrapped up in p-values. The most important determinant should be the effect size. The effect size chosen should be realistic; too large an effect size is the same as being too optimistic about the size of the association – as an absurd example, would we assume a treatment will add 60 years to a patient's life expectancy? Too small an effect size not only can result in an impractically large sample size but also assumes the effect of interest is negligible. On the other hand, consider designing a study where you want to show that two effects are the same within some boundary – the boundary should be reasonably tight! This gets back to the discussion of the confidence interval in the previous chapter.

You can also improve statistical power by appropriate selection of a study population. For example, you could focus on patients who are believed more likely to benefit from a treatment, so the expected difference will be higher, which will increase the effect size. Restricting the patient population has the risk that your resulting population may be too distinct from the normal patient pool for the results to be usefully generalizable.

A two-tailed t-test divides the Type I error into equal, recognizing that if a Type I error does occur, it may appear as one group being falsely measured as either larger or smaller than the other. A one-tailed test is predicated on only a change in one direction being of interest, either an increase or a decrease. Looking back in Figure 2.1, we could be asking if our 5% chance of Type I error was shared between both tails or only in one tail. For example, if you are testing whether a new method performs better than an existing method, then "not better" contains both "worse" and "no difference." You can justify a smaller sample size for a statistical test, with the caveat that if you've bet on a change in one direction and the data shows a large change in the other, it's a dubious practice to change to a two-tailed test and claim that the "wrong direction" change is statistically significant. Abelson [2] points out that this is essentially a "one-and-a-half-tailed test" with an effective Type I error rate of 7.5% – 0.05 in the one-tailed test your study was powered for, and 0.025 in the second tail you've snuck in!

The preceding descriptions assume you are in the relatively simple situation of comparing two groups. Comparisons between three or more groups can be a little more complicated. For hypothesis tests, it is possible to treat a category with N levels as being $N * (N - 1)$ multiple tests, which will give you a reasonable sample size estimate using a correction for inflated Type I error. Adjusting for multiple tests gets us into math outside the sphere of this book, but the simplest possible adjustment is the Bonferroni adjustment: if you have M tests, then your significance threshold is p-value less than $0.05/M$, so the total error of the tests sums up to 0.05. This is echoed in the two-tailed statistical test, where there are essentially two statistical tests – one for a positive change and one for a negative change. If all of the possible tests are not of interest, then you can use a smaller adjustment, but you should confine the analysis only to those specific tests. Similarly, a study testing multiple endpoints may want to divide up Type I error among endpoints to reduce the risk of inflated Type I error. The Holm-Bonferroni adjustment is a more lenient version; if you have M tests, you compare your smallest p-value against $0.05/M$ and if it is significant, you compare your next smallest against $0.05/(M - 1)$ and keep going until you reach a p-value that is not significant or you've done all M tests.

Stopping a clinical study early because the results are particularly promising or are looking futile is another example of doing multiple testing. You would test once at a planned point and again at the end of the study. However, the issues are complicated and still being debated. This is an example of a statistical project you shouldn't try on your own – consult an expert. As a general rule, even if the short-term results look good, remember the Law of Large Numbers and wait until the end. (Of course, if the results are immediate and spectacular in your specific case, don't feel bound by general rules – but get a second opinion anyway!)

Many statistics classes will teach the method of starting with an *omnibus* test such as an ANOVA to determine whether there is any difference at all among three or more categories and then applying a pairwise test to see where the statistically significant differences may be found. You can estimate sample size for the ANOVA, but you might find you do not have enough power to show pairwise differences. On the other hand, you can start by planning pairwise comparisons between groups and base your sample size on that. An advantage of "skipping" the ANOVA this way may be that some comparisons may not be important, interesting, or useful and so you recoup statistical power by not having to do them.

If your goal is to show that two groups are in fact equivalent, then you want to calculate sample size based on creating a sufficiently tight estimate for the difference between groups. That requires clinical insight as well as mathematics because the CI should be within the bounds for which the observed difference would be clinically negligible. However, we would like to point out here that the p-value adjustment for multiple testing would not be appropriate in this case for the paradoxical reason that a tighter threshold for a significant finding would make it more difficult to demonstrate that two groups are in fact different, which would disprove your argument for equivalence. As a general rule, try to avoid design decisions where a critic could argue that you've made it easier to demonstrate the result you wanted to show.

For a study using regressions with continuous predictors (age, weight, etc.), one more consideration may be the range of values for the predictor [27, 28]. For example, if you're interested in how age affects outcome, you would be better off with data where age is distributed among a wider range, say, 40–80 years instead of 50–60 years. Mathematically, the regression slope over the range of a predictor (age, time, etc.) increases as the range increases and as there are more values at the extremes of the range [27]. Bland and Altman [28] show an example of outcome versus BMI where the four correlations within BMI ranges (underweight, normal, overweight, obese) are each smaller than the correlation over the entire range of BMI.

Analysis of events, such as that done with logistic regression, requires a different approach. You should base statistical power on the number of events you expect to observe, which is a function of both the rate of the event and the number of patients. A historical rule of thumb suggests that you will want 10–20 events per parameter being studied [27, 29]. That's per parameter, not per variable, as a category with M levels will have M-1 parameters. A recent sophisticated study of sample size calculations [30] describes how the sample size used can impact not only the precision of the estimate but also the generalizability of the resulting statistical model to a new data set. Note that this is for creating a predictive model. Being able to show that a particular parameter contributes meaningfully is a different question. The G*Power3 software does offer tools to get an idea of the sample size for logistic or Poisson regression (discussed in Chapter 12) so you can design a study to test parameter values. For a very complicated situation, the best approach may be simulations: generate artificial data similar to what you expect to see in the study, changing sample sizes, and determine at what N you get acceptable levels of Type II error (false negatives). If you're at that level of complication, you should already be collaborating with a statistician.

Statisticians are often asked to do a power analysis after the data has been collected. The value of such post-hoc analysis is debatable. For the study being done, the data has already been collected. A power analysis done before data collection tells you how much data is adequate for your planned analysis, though it may not be useful if you either have a very small data set already (say, for a rare condition) or a very large database where it costs nothing to use all of it. After the study, a power analysis can indicate whether a non-significant test might have been significant with a larger data set, but a confidence interval may be a better indicator of whether you had a potentially meaningful finding lurking somewhere in your statistically indeterminate results. Possibly the best use of a post-hoc power analysis would be to plan a study that would be more definitive. (Whether any study can be completely definitive is a very interesting question. ...)

At the end of this section, we should acknowledge the researcher who is trying to plan an analysis of a small data set. Although nothing actually prevents you from applying any particular statistical tool, your best option might not be technical at all: network! If other people interested in the topic are also looking at small sets of data at their end, then there may be a productive collaboration based on pooled data. Publication of a small study can be valuable. The Cochrane Collaboration, which is a standard for meta-analysis and systematic reviews, based their emblem on the results of a meta-analysis of studies evaluating giving corticosteroids to women about to give birth prematurely; individual studies were not statistically significant, but the pooled evidence indicated that the steroids could save the premature baby.

CHAPTER 6

Showing the Data to Yourself First – Graphs and Tables, Part 1

I N CHAPTER 15, WE will discuss the best ways to present your analyses at the conclusion of the study. At this point, it is appropriate to discuss how to look at the data that is going into the statistical analyses. It is looking at the x-rays and lab findings before operating. You need to know before applying a statistical test whether the data is consistent with the assumptions of the test. You need to know if any variable suffers from inconsistent coding, unusual values, or missing data. You may discover that the relationship between predictor and outcome is more complicated than you thought it was – perhaps it has a U shape, or perhaps it seems to depend on the value of another variable. John Tukey has said, "The greatest value of a picture is when it forces us to notice what we never expected to see."

Also, you may have heard colleagues say that they will often have the paper largely written before they even begin collecting data. This is a reasonable approach, as it helps organize thinking, as long as you are willing to rewrite the paper when unexpected results come in. But it also obliges the author to consider what sort of tables and graphs should be included and how they can tell the story.

A table is convenient in many ways. It can contain as many rows and columns as required. The reader can get exact values from it. Readability can be improved by shading rows or columns, bolding text, and adding headings. However, it becomes harder to compare groups or spot trends.

A histogram of values makes it immediately apparent if data is symmetric or skewed and if different groups seem to have different distributions. Whether an apparent difference can be systematic or explainable by simple randomness is a matter for statistical testing. The histogram also makes it possible to assess whether transforming the data results in something closer to a Gaussian distribution. For example, lognormal distribution (Figure 2.1C) is defined as a distribution where the raw data is skewed but the logarithm of values is Gaussian.

A histogram is a familiar option for showing a distribution graphically – it comes installed in Excel. Another option is a boxplot, also known as a box-and-whisker, which is standard in most statistical packages but can be done "by hand" in Excel with minor effort. The box is defined by the 25% and 75% quartiles of the data's distribution and is bisected by the median of the distribution. The whiskers extend from the box toward the minimum and maximum of the data. Both the histogram and the boxplot make it possible to spot extreme values, which may need to be addressed in the analysis. Methods for doing so are considered in Chapter 7.

Of course, you can also describe the distribution in a table – or the main text of the manuscript. Whether you use mean or median depends on the distribution and the message of your study. Even for a skewed distribution, an arithmetic mean can give useful information such as blood milliliters transfused per patient. Standard deviation and variance do not have their intuitively useful meanings – 95% of values being within 2 standard deviations of the mean, for example, if the distribution is not Gaussian but it may still be useful to quantify the variation in the data. Using interquartile range (25% and 75% quartiles) instead of variance substitutes two numbers for one, but it does usefully describe the variability in a skewed distribution.

For a categorical variable, you will be tabulating or plotting the rate at which the variable has each of its possible values. For a binary variable, it's usually sufficient to show the rate for one value, such as whether the patient is female or has a complication. Bar plots and tables become useful if the variable has multiple categories or if you are comparing rates of a particular value among two or more groups, or both. Although you can calculate confidence intervals on the rate estimates, consider whether it's useful to present. On the one hand, it helps to keep in mind that the observed rate is not the same thing as the underlying probability generating the observations. On the other, you have a finite opportunity to hold the reader's focus; why distract them by answering questions they would not need to ask?

Use pie charts at your own discretion. Many data analysts hate them. The main limitation of a pie chart is that only one statement can be made: that one or two categories make up the largest shares of the distribution. If that's enough for you to say, a pie chart may be adequate, although you might still consider alternatives. The pie chart won't make it easy to compare rates directly against each other unless each pie slice is labelled with the actual value, and then you've sacrificed the relative simplicity that makes the pie chart appealing. There's also no way to describe the margin of error. Where looking at the detail is important, use a bar chart or a line plot.

Plotting data against time can reveal whether some numbers show a gradual change over the years or over seasons. It can also show whether a change in practice (say, perhaps a change in coding or diagnoses for a condition) causes a sharp change in recorded data. This is important because a statistical test will ask, in essence, "All things being equal, how does this predictor affect the outcome?" You can simplify your task by focusing your analysis on periods when all things can be shown or assumed to be equal.

This brings us to another comparison of graphs and tables. A table can be good for multiple comparisons as long as all the columns fit on the page. Graphs are good for making visual comparisons between trends, but after about five lines or so in the figure the graph can become confusing.

You might think of there being a division of labor between statistical tests and presenting data in graphs or tables. An association between variables can be detected in a statistical test without necessarily being visible to the eye. Similarly, a finding in a graph or a table might be striking to the eye, but the statistical test would not be able to exclude the possibility that the apparent relationship is a simple chance.

Figure 6.1 shows an example of how looking at graphs under different situations can make you aware of issues. The graphed data is from a study of outcomes in kidney stone surgery [31] and is considered a classic example of Simpson's paradox. The study looked at the success rates for open and percutaneous surgery in small and large (or multiple) stones. We cut off the Y-axis at 50% so the proportion of failures would be clearer. On the left, we look at the percentages of success and failure using a stacked bar chart, with the Y-axis cut at 50% for improved visibility. On the top, we have the surgeries subdivided by the size of the stones; on the bottom we have the surgeries pooled. What's striking is that although you can tell in the top plot that percutaneous surgeries have more failures than open surgeries for both the small and large/multiple stones, when you look at the bottom plot, it appears as though the open surgeries have a higher rate of failures.

The paradox is explained by looking at the right column, which shows the numbers. For small stones, more percutaneous

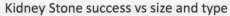

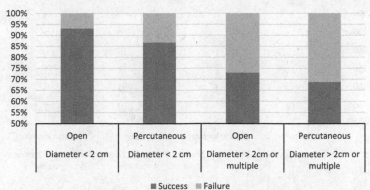

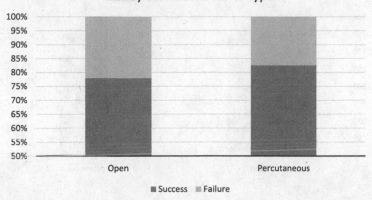

FIGURE 6.1 Visible results can depend on shifts in scale and on the control for other variables. This is a classic example where percutaneous surgery had higher failures than open surgery in both high- and low-diameter groups but lower failures overall. This was a consequence of not only the actual success rate of the surgeries but the numbers of surgeries done.

operations were done. For large stones, more open surgeries were done. So the pooled data is not appropriately weighted to show what is really going on.

A purist such as Edward Tufte would point out that in most circumstances, we do not want stacked plots. As with the pie

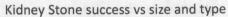

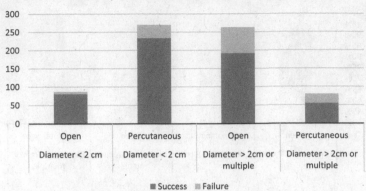

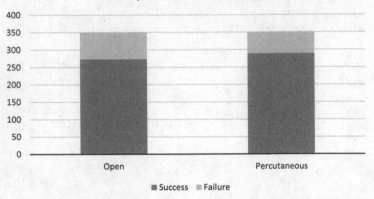

FIGURE 6.2 Three scenarios for a continuous outcome showing the need to control for an interaction in order to accurately describe the data.

chart, it is difficult to show any margin of error. However, using stacked plots in this context, including plotting the same data multiple ways, helps us understand the data.

A similar reason to plot data with sub-categories is shown in Figure 6.2. On the top plot, we have a relatively simple case that one curve is simply offset from another by a constant amount. If we were setting this up as a regression equation, we would use $Y = A*X + B_{group}$, where B_{group} could take on multiple values based on group membership. The middle plot and bottom plots both show cases where the slope depends on group membership. The regression equation would look something like $Y = A_{group}*X + B_{group}$ either way. But if we simply did a correlation between Y and X, we might falsely conclude in the bottom plot that there was no relationship on average, as the two groups have opposite slopes.

CHAPTER 7

How Normal Is a Gaussian Distribution? What to Do with Extreme Values?

NON-GAUSSIAN DISTRIBUTIONS

In theory, probability distributions can be spikier than the Gaussian, flatter, have multiple peaks, or be biased toward higher or lower values. There are tests for whether a variable is truly Gaussian, but these have the usual issues with statistical tests: for a small data set, they may not be able to state whether a distribution is Gaussian; for a large data set, even small deviations may be statistically significant; and there is still the question of whether the deviation is large enough to be meaningful.

In practice, the exception you are most likely to see will be a right-skewed distribution, where lower values are more common and the median is less than the mean. The most intuitive example of such a distribution is salaries, where most make lower salaries and only a few make the highest. Count data, including salaries, usually follows such a distribution. Other possible examples are operative times, lengths of stay in hospital, or some lab values. The particular problem with such a distribution is that the variance will increase with the mean, so a small fluctuation at small values has the same probability as a large fluctuation at larger values.

A potential fix is to apply an appropriate mathematical function to the data so that the resulting transformed data will be less skewed and more Gaussian. Although the square root and the reciprocal (1/X) can be used, the most convenient transformation is usually the logarithm. Some statistical packages will have a Box-Cox transformation tool, which will give you a range of simple transformations. What makes the logarithm convenient is that log (A times B) equals log(A) plus log(B). A t-test or regression will assume that predictors are adding or subtracting to a baseline value. If you do a t-test or regression on the logarithm of the outcome and apply the appropriate back-transformation on the parameters, then your results are in terms of multipliers – 1.2 for a 20% increase, for example, or 0.8 for a 20% decrease. This falls out of the math: if $\log(Y)$ is modelled as $A + Bx$, then Y is assumed to follow $\exp(A)*\exp(B)^x$, so if $\exp(B)$ is 1.2, then two units' increase in X multiplies Y by $1.2^2 = 1.44$.

The logarithmic transform is a helpful trick for skewed data with two caveats. One is that if you back-transform, you do not actually get the expected value (conditional mean), although if you assume the log-transformed data had a symmetric distribution, then you can assume the back-transformed prediction is the median. The other warning is that if you're using Excel, be careful that the log function is the base 10 logarithm whose inverse transform is 10^x, or 10 raised to the power of x, while the LN function is the natural log and the corresponding inverse transform is $\exp(x)$. Getting the two confused will not affect statistical significance testing, but it will distort estimates of differences between groups.

Also, don't make decisions based purely on mathematical convenience. For example, supposing our interest was in was how quickly something was done, such as a timed test to get out of a chair. By definition, speed is distance divided by time. In that case, we would want to explore using either time or 1/time as our outcome measurement.

EXTREME VALUES

Applying statistics accurately means being aware of the data. For example, the mean is based on summing up all the values in the set and dividing it by the size of the set, so it may be affected by unusually large or small values. Because the standard deviation (SD) is based on the average squared difference between the mean and every measurement in the data set, it can be even more affected by outliers than the mean. Imagine combining two populations, one with a mean of 5 and one with a mean of 10. If they make up equal proportions, the combined mean is $(0.5 \times 5) + (0.5 \times 10) = 7.5$. If the group with the smaller mean makes up 80% of the combination, then the combined average is $(0.8 \times 5) + (0.2 \times 10) = 6$. The mean calculated from a set of data is an estimate of the expected value of the distribution. Now assume there's a third group with a mean of 100 (an outlier!), and it makes up 1% of the combination. Then, if we have $(0.8 \times 5) + (0.19 \times 10) + (0.01 \times 100)$, the combined mean is $4 + 1.9 + 1 = 6.9$. If the outsized group had a mean of 1,000, the combined mean would be 15.9.

The *median* is an example of a more robust way of describing data. The median is simply the value where 50% of the data is above and 50% is below. In a normal distribution, which is symmetric, the average (mean) and the median are the same value, as the distribution is just as likely to be above the mean as below it. Imagine two studies of incomes among randomly-selected individuals, and one of those samples includes Bill Gates. The mean wealth of Gates' group will probably be much larger than that of the other group, but the median wealth will be comparable. In our artificial examples before, with the combined means of 6, 5.9, or 15.9, the median should be close to 5, although the exact values depend on the distributions of the data. This is a disadvantage of the median – it's not as friendly to simple mathematics as the mean. Another difference between the mean and the median is that the median is not necessarily the expected value for a member of the population. For a symmetric distribution such as the Gaussian, the mean should equal the median, but this would not be true for a skewed (off-center) distribution.

The symmetry of the Gaussian distribution often allows for the spotting of non-normal data from a published summary table. By the mathematical definition of the Gaussian distribution, 95% of the observed values will be within 2 SD of the mean. Thus, if you see a variable where the SD is larger than half the mean, and where the number is not expected to have negative values (like most physical measurements), the data was likely not normal. Another giveaway is if a range is given, and it is not symmetric around the mean or the median. In these cases, although the means and SD can still contain useful information about typical values and variation, they may not be the best descriptors and statistical tests assuming that normality may not be the most informative, either.

There are two possible explanations for extreme values or outliers. One is that this is the result of normal variation. A Gaussian distribution will have some fraction of very low or very high values, and a Poisson distribution will tend to have many lower values and fewer high ones. You can check this by graphing data and changing your axis to logarithmic. This is shown in Figure 7.1, where the same X and Y are graphed using linear and logarithmic axes: in both cases, there is a visible relationship, but the logarithmic transform makes it clearer. You may also have naturally atypical patients: a study of obesity effects may be thrown off by including wrestlers or football players among an otherwise non-athletic population.

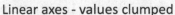

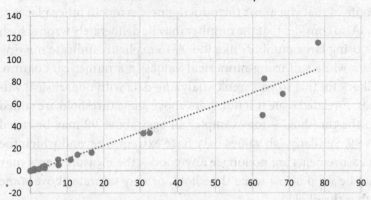

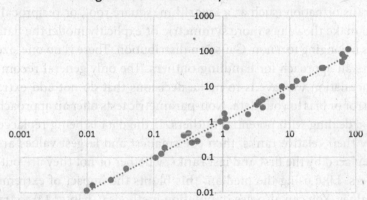

FIGURE 7.1   What appear to be clumped values on a linear axis show an even distribution on a log axis. Apparent outliers may be a consequence of the scale used.

The other possibility for outliers is that there was a recording error and the number is simply wrong. In that case, unless you can go back and confirm or correct the outlier, you may have to drop the outlier and treat the value as missing data. In some cases, you may be able to apply a common-sense rule for restoring dropped decimal points, converting occasional uses of inches into centimeters, and so on, but investigate before applying to confirm that you aren't introducing new errors in other places.

Also consider that the number may be deliberately wrong, such as using large numbers like 99999 to explicitly indicate missing data while still using numerical values in a numerical column. Check for that so you aren't analyzing data with nonsensical values. A related issue is if numbers above some threshold are coded to the threshold – for example, all ages above 99 may be saved as 99. Similarly, lab values may have extremes beyond which the measurements are no longer any good – the measurements may not be valid below some threshold, or may saturate above some other threshold.

Depending on the needs of the study, it may be appropriate to exclude the most extreme values, apply some mathematical transformation (such as a logarithm, square root, or reciprocal) to make the values more symmetric or explicitly model the data as belonging to a non-Gaussian distribution. There is no one size fits all approach for handling outliers. The only general recommendation we have is to make decisions that do not add extra error or bias to your data. Non-parametric tests offer an approach for dealing with potential outliers. If the data is being replaced by their relative ranks, then the smallest and largest values are replaced by the first and last ranks, whether or not they are outliers. Like using the median, this blunts the impact of extreme values. You can also use imputation methods (Chapter 14) to try to replace the outliers with plausible values.

ORDINAL DATA

When we see numbers such as 1, 2, 3, 4, 5 ... we expect two things. One is that they occur in sequence: 1 before 2, 2 before 3, and so on. The other is that there are equal steps. Going from 1 to 2 is the same interval as from 3 to 4 or 5 to 6.

Ordinal data requires a special approach because even though the ordering is present, the interval assumption is not true. For example, we may ask a patient to answer a questionnaire from

one of five choices: "Strongly disagree," "Disagree," "No opinion," "Agree," "Strongly Agree." Can we expect that the step from
"Strongly disagree" to "Disagree" is the same as from "Agree"
to "Strongly Disagree?" What about steps on either side of "No
opinion?"

Questionnaires aren't the only such source of ordinal data. The
American Spinal Injury Association (ASIA) scale for spinal cord
injury is A through E. The American Society of Anethesiologists
(ASA) scale is numerical, but the numbers represent categories:
1 for healthy, 2 for mild systemic disease, 3 for severe systemic
disease, and so on.

Of course, it's always possible to treat ordinal values as numbers and take an average and a standard deviation; it's done all
the time, and nothing stops us. But is that the best way to go?

One alternative approach is to simply collapse categories so
the ordinal scale becomes a binary one: did the patient improve,
was the patient satisfied, and so on – then apply the appropriate
methods for the analysis of binary outcomes. But now information is beinnstiog thrown out: if we recode our earlier example
into "agree yes or no," then we lose any distinction between
"Agree" and "Strongly Agree" or between "Strongly Disagree"
and "No opinion." We could try repeating the binary analysis
shifting the point of division, but now we have four analyses of
our five-level outcome, blurring the outcome a different way each
time. A chi-squared test comparing categories seems reasonable,
but that throws out the ordering information.

Many of you have probably seen non-parametric equivalents
to common statistical tools (see Box). These tests become "non-
parametric" because they are based on ranks of data and so do
not assume any distribution. For ordinal data, we already begin
with ranked data, so the non-parametric tests are ideally suited
for dealing with ordinal data. The parametric tests in the left column are called parametric because they try to estimate parameters for both the process of interest (factors contributing to the
outcome) and the random variation (or rather, that variation that

can't be explained by the predictors included in the analysis). If the wrong test is selected, the parameters estimated may be misleading; we will get into these issues in Chapter 11.

Parametric test (assumes Gaussian distribution)	Non-parametric (rank-based) equivalent
T-test	Mann–Whitney or Wilcoxon
ANOVA	Kruskal–Wallis or Friedman
Correlation	Spearman's rho or Kendall's tau

CHAPTER 8

All Probabilities Are Conditional

"CONDITIONAL PROBABILITY" MAY BE a term some readers have heard. The notation P(A|B) is math shorthand read aloud "Probability of A given B," which means the probability of observing event A given that we have also observed event B. If A and B have nothing to do with each other, then P(A|B) is equal to P(A), the overall probability of event A. The p-value is a conditional probability, where A is the chance of observing a test statistic of a certain value or greater and B is the condition where the null hypothesis is true and the results are just due to random variations.

It's been observed that all probabilities are conditional. For example, the probability that a patient with hip surgery will need a revision is the probability of needing a revision conditional on having hip surgery, P(Revision|Surgery). This may seem nonsensical at first – why would a patient need a revision if they haven't had surgery? However, the total probability that anyone on the street will need a revision is the product P(Revision|Surgery) *P(Surgery), which is the probability of the person having the surgery. Similarly, even an analysis of the entire patient population seen by a health system is conditional on the patient belonging to the health system – although, for a large and diverse population, it is usually reasonable to assume the results are generalizable.

Bayes' theorem states that you can calculate $P(B|A)$ as $P(A|B) * P(B)/P(A)$. You have probably already seen sensitivity and positive predictive value in studies of diagnostic tests; Bayes' theorem links them. Sensitivity is the conditional probability $P(+|D)$, where "+" means that a test is positive and D means that a patient has a disease. The positive predictive value is $P(D|+)$ or the probability that the patient actually has a disease, given a positive result. The relationship between them is the ratio between $P(D)$ and $P(+)$. $P(D)$ is simply the prevalence of the disease, and $P(+)$ is easy to calculate from the prevalence, the sensitivity, and the specificity. The false-positive rate is 1 – specificity, and the chance of not having the disease is 1 – prevalence, so $P(+)$ = prevalence * sensitivity + (1 – prevalance) * (1 – specificity). Hopefully you're already aware of the caveat with the sensitivity that a positive test for a rare condition can have a low positive predictive value.

Let's look at this in terms of the study that would have been used to estimate sensitivity and specificity. The study would have N subjects, where TP and TN are true positive and true negative, FP and FN are false positive and false negative, and N = TP + FP + FN + TN. The total number of patients with the disease is TP + FN, and the total probability of having the disease in the study population is [TP + FN]/N. The total number of the people who tested positive is TP + FP, and the probability of a positive test result in the population is [TP + FP]/N. Sensitivity is estimated as the positives across all patients who had the disease, TP/[TP + FN], and the positive predictive value is those who had the disease across all positives, TP/[TP + FP]. Bayes' theorem states that $P(B|A)$ is $P(A|B) * P(B)/P(A)$ so the positive predictive value should be the sensitivity times the total probability of having the disease divided by the total probability of testing positive, or TP/[TP + FP] = TP/[TP + FN] * [TP + FN]/N * N/[TP + FP]. The Ns cancel. We can also see why high sensitivity can still result in a low predictive value. If the false positives are high compared to the false negatives, then the positive predictive value will be low compared to specificity.

Keep in mind that these sensitivities and specificities calculated in the study are statistical estimates and as such have some margin of error. The standard error for a proportion p estimated from a sample N is sqrt(p*(1 − p)/N), and the 95% confidence interval for the estimate is p ± 1.96 times the standard error. If your study includes 100 patients with the condition (TP + FN) and your observed sensitivity is 0.9 (TP = 90 patients), then the standard error is sqrt (0.9 * 0.1/100) = 0.03, and your confidence interval is 0.84–0.96.

We already pointed out that the p-value is a conditional probability; the chance of getting the observed test statistic is higher if the null hypothesis of no association is true. We define an acceptable upper limit on apparently significant test statistics over all possible test statistics when the null hypothesis is true, which we could imagine as FP/[FP + TN], or 1 − specificity, being under 0.05. In this case, FP is when the test statistic is significant and the null hypothesis is true, and TP is when the test statistic is significant and the null hypothesis is false. Similarly, statistical power is a declaration that we want TP/[TP + FN], or the rate of significant test statistics over all possible test statistics when the null hypothesis is false, to be at least some high rate, typically 80%. But where we could calculate positive and negative predictive values for diagnostic tests, having TP, TN, FP, and FN at our fingertips, we can't do the same to estimate the probability that the null hypothesis is true or false based on our data, at least, not under the frequentist framework generally used.

What's called Bayesian statistics uses Bayes' theorem to update an initial estimate on the parameter estimates (difference between groups, slope of a regression, etc.) based on the data. If the assumed prior distribution of parameter estimates is P(Θ), then the updated distribution of parameter values given the observed data is P(Θ |Data). Bayesian approaches to statistics can demand a lot of computing power, so they have become practical and increasingly popular as computer technology improves. The differences between the Bayesian and the frequentist views arise from differences in defining probability in the first place and are beyond the scope of this book. However, reading up on this debate is recommended. Google "frequentist vs. Bayesian" and take a few sips from the resulting flood.

CHAPTER 9

Quality versus Quantity in Data

KNOW WHAT YOU'RE GETTING

Although anecdotes are not to be confused with studies of very small sample size, there are a few anecdotes from Dr. Maltenfort's experience that illustrate how statistical sophistication, at any level, is at the mercy of the data actually provided.

Dr. Maltenfort was doing an analysis of stroke outcomes. One of the potential predictors was smoking. But something funny was going on: smokers were associated with better stroke outcomes. Dr. Maltenfort spent a few days going around in circles, trying different statistical models and different sets of predictors, trying to explain what was going wrong by trying more and different analyses. Then, he gave up and asked one of the neurosurgeons whether there might be an issue with the data that might explain the problem. The explanation was that the smoking habits of the patient were assessed on discharge, not on admission. If the patient wasn't capable of answering questions about smoking, they weren't marked as a smoker. The good news was that this explained the problem; the bad news was that the relationship between smoking and stroke was biased in this data; no analysis method would be able to disentangle it.

Another stroke surgeon wanted to do a study looking at readmission rates in patients who had been operated on for aneurysms. Successful patients would be the ones who never came back. Dr. Maltenfort asked how he was going to track patients who had died after discharge since they presumably couldn't be counted as successes. That was the end of the project.

Lastly, there was a potentially excellent study on stroke outcomes where the data had been collected before talking to any statistician. There is a famous, dreadful, and yet truthful wisecrack from the famous statistician Ronald Fisher that this can be equivalent to asking the statistician for an autopsy to discover what the study died of. The demographics table was accurate and detailed, along with the table for patient status on admission, the table for treatments, and the table for outcomes. The only thing missing was a key to link the individual tables together for a comprehensive analysis.

Of the scenarios reviewed above, only the third could have been addressed technically – by adding an appropriate field to make the linkage of the tables possible. The other two could only be addressed by appropriate planning for collecting useful data. Hence, the quality of the data is more important than the quantity of the data. While it may not be possible to correct the quality of the data, there are methods that can help maintain data in a useful format. There is an excellent review (one might say "manifesto") of these principles available online called *Tidy Data* by Hadley Wickham [32]. It is recommended reading, but it is also written from a general perspective, not a clinical one. The important take-home is that before beginning data collection, think about how it may be analyzed and presented.

PROPER LAYOUT

If you are getting data directly from your institutional database, it is probably already organized in a usable format. We say "probably" because the data may still require review and cleaning. (We discussed the potential issues with outliers and skewed distributions in Chapter 7.) Certain rules are likely to be followed:

- Each column contains a single variable. It might be age, gender, the presence of comorbidity, and so on.

- Each row is a single record. What that record is will depend on the nature of the data. It may be per patient, per visit, or per surgery.

- Each variable has a single value for a given row and column.

- Values within a column are all of the same type. That one can be particularly tricky with lab values where you can go from numbers to "< detection threshold."

The data may also come in Excel format. This is not automatically a bad thing. Unfortunately, Excel offers a few features aimed at making the data more readable to humans that will introduce problems for importing into a statistical program. Hidden rows/columns or colored text will mean nothing to the program. Similarly, it is easy to type all comorbidities as a list in a single column. Again, the program will be "asthma, rheumatism" and not see any overlap with patients whose sole comorbidity is "asthma" or "rheumatism." Similarly, Excel may not see "Asthma," "asthma," and "Asthma" with a space as a different text, but another program may be pickier. In other programs, "Y," "y," "Yes," "YES," and "yes" may all be interpreted as different variables; thus consistent formatting is imperative. Excel may save a percentage as a decimal, which is 75% as 0.75; if the column isn't consistent with using the percentage sign, then 50% will be saved as 0.5 and 50 will be saved as 50.

To provide a consistent data format for the ease of data analysis, it may be beneficial to code variables. For example, coding all patient comorbidities, setting up multiple columns of different comorbidities (e.g. diabetes, myocardial infarction, asthma), and delineating if each comorbidity is present or not, with "0" for not present and "1" for present, are a clear method of describing if a comorbidity is present instead of listing all comorbidities. It is also better to present laboratory values with the same units and just list the numbers within the datasheet for the ease of statistical analysis.

For longitudinal data where each patient may be recorded more than once, say, at regular intervals post-operatively, you may need to decide between *long* and *wide* formats. If you follow the "tidy data" rules, then most software packages offer easy tools to transition between formats once you've collected the data, but you still have to collect the data the first time. Say you measure patient weight once a month for six months. A wide-format file would have one column for patient identifier and six columns for weights, one for each month. A long-format file would have one column for patient identifier, one column for months and one column for weights. The patient identifier would be seen in six different rows, each one numbered 1 to 6 in the month column. A long format has certain advantages if you don't measure the patients at consistent intervals: perhaps this patient has measurements at 1.5, 5, and 7 months, and that patient has measurements at 2 and 6 months. But for some statistical tests or plots, say, of the first month's weight versus the last month's weight, you need to put the data in wide format. An advantage of a long format is it can be more compact, but if you have to transition to a wide format, you will probably have a situation where not every patient has a measurement at every time. In that case, your options may be to let the cells be empty or to fill in a value such as zero; filling in with zero would be sensible if you were looking at counts of events where empty cells meant no events but would not be sensible for data such as weight. Be careful with data manipulations, so you don't inadvertently plug in erroneous values!

When setting up data to be analyzed, remember that computers have very little intelligence, artificial or otherwise. What they can do are a number of repetitive tasks in an organized way that produce overall sophisticated behavior. We will make no representation of whether statisticians are any smarter. We can advise that consistency is always good, and ambiguity is always bad.

TO CATEGORIZE OR NOT TO CATEGORIZE

One of the strongest general rules for handling data is that you should never force a continuous variable into categories unless there is a compelling reason to do so [33]. First, we will review why you shouldn't dichotomize data, and then we will discuss why you may want to do so.

The major argument against is that information is lost at the point of the split. Perhaps you want to look at patients on either side of 65 years old. Patients younger than 65 will include those who are 35 and who are 64. Patients older than 65 will include those who are 66 and who are 96. By lumping broad groups together, you've added noise to the problem. Then, you have to justify the cut point selected. Yes, you could try using multiple categories, say under 45, 45–65, and over 65. You're still risking some information loss, plus which you've now cost yourself in a new area: binary variables, like continuous variables, only require one parameter to define them. If you have a category with M values, you need M − 1 parameters, as one category becomes a reference level. Note that a binary variable has M = 2. Then, you have more cut-points to justify. Of course, basing divisions on percentiles (medians, quartiles, etc.) has the advantage that you have groups of equal size and ordered by magnitude, but that doesn't necessarily mean that the percentile cut-off has clinical relevance. And if you are using one set of breakpoints and another researcher is using a different set, someone reading both papers will have a harder time trying to assess whether the results of both papers are consistent.

One of the major reasons for converting a continuous number into categories is that you want to plot or tabulate results. If you are plotting treatment versus outcome controlling for age, for example, then you have to convert continuous age into discrete levels. For plots, you can flip things around and plot age versus outcome with subgroups based on a variable that is already categorical. That won't work for tables.

Another possible reason to categorize is the assumption that there is a linear (straight-line) relationship between predictor and outcome. However, that is not necessarily true. For example, health risks might arise from being either underweight or overweight. One approach is to convert to categories, for example, the Centers for Disease Control and Prevention (CDC) cut-points for BMI as underweight, normal, overweight, or obese. For a statistical model, a better approach would be to use a polynomial fit where we would have the outcome as a function of BMI, BMI^2, and BMI^3. The polynomial would capture the nonlinearity and allow for a more precise estimation of how the predictor is associated with the outcome. The polynomial has a more sophisticated relative known as the spline, which allows very complicated nonlinearities to be fit, at the cost of not being able to specifically describe parameters associated with the fit. For numerical reasons, if you use a polynomial, you may want to center the variable by subtracting out BMI. One reason to center variables is that large differences in extreme values can introduce numerical issues that will cause your software to complain about potential inaccuracies being introduced. For example, suppose BMI goes from 15 to 40 with a mean of 20 and then the extremes of BMI^2 are 25 to 1,600 and BMI^3, 3,375 to 64,000. For $BMI_0 = BMI - 20$ (ranging from -5 to $+20$), the extremes of BMI_0^2 are 25 to 400 and BMI^3, -125 to 8,000. Another reason to center variables is that the results may be more intuitive if you can discuss changes relative to the average patient rather than relative to zero.

There is also the desire to establish a clinical threshold for making decisions such as when or how to treat a patient or whether a patient is high or low risk. However, as discussed in other areas of this book, such thresholds would be based on noisy estimates. A threshold for treatment or diagnostic decision might be viewed as skeptically as $p < 0.05$ for statistical significance. Giannoni et al. [34] offer a detailed review of pitfalls in trying to assess such thresholds. One we would emphasize here is that the threshold that's valid for one group of patients may not be valid for another, based on age or comorbidities.

Practical Examples

EXAMPLE 1: BLOOD LOSS

Imagine we want to investigate blood loss in surgeries. That seems simple enough. Excessive blood loss endangers the patient. If we have a measurement for blood loss, then we can use regression to estimate the expected blood loss. The more we look at the details of planning a study, however, the more complications we encounter.

First off, how do we measure blood loss? There is no agreed-upon "gold standard" approach. Direct methods include using suction canisters or weighing sponges. There are also several equations [35] for estimating blood loss from patient measurements such as body surface area (estimated) and from pre-op and post-op laboratory measurements such as hemoglobin or hematocrit, but, of course, different equations yield different results. And if the equation gives something that looks ridiculous – say, a negative blood loss – the temptation will be to throw out that data point. Except then you may bias your results because the "ridiculous" value is affected by the noise in your measurements and regression models will try to estimate the noise as well as the predictive parameters.

The methods used for measuring data will affect the choices for analysis. If you are using an equation based on the patient body surface area, you may want to think twice about using body mass index (BMI) as a predictor, as heavier patients should have a higher body surface area; you'd be using a predictor that was already part of your outcome. Transfusions received by the patient would affect the post-operative lab results but not the blood loss from direct measurement. Then again, perhaps you want to predict the need for transfusions, perhaps to estimate demand on blood banks, so we would use transfusion units as an outcome, but that introduces two new issues, one being that the decision to transfuse can vary from surgeon to surgeon, another being that the outcome has changed from blood loss as a continuous-valued number to the number of transfusion units, which might be 0, 1, 2, etc. Accounting for surgeon variation or for small integer counts would require different methods. You could, for example, address surgeon variation with a random effect for the surgeon and transfusion unit counts with either a count-data model or an ordinal regression model.

Also, consider how much blood loss is excessive. The level of blood loss which introduces health risks is probably more than the median or mean blood loss per patient; otherwise, these risks would be a routine part of the surgery. There are studies of how much blood loss is acceptable, but they depend on subjective choices by the patient of what post-operative lab values are acceptable. You could use some arbitrary percentile for blood loss – for example, 75% or 95% – and look at what factors affect the risk of a patient crossing that threshold; that's arbitrary, but you could always try running different models with different percentiles. You could also create a new model from available data looking at the risk of poor outcomes using blood loss as a predictor and using the new model results as a guide, but the new model results might be affected by what other factors were included or left out in the predictor set.

Simple questions can have complicated answers. This is where advice from Tukey comes back into play. For the sample question of what impacts blood loss, there is a range of approximate

answers. Based on the information at hand or the needs moti-
vating the study, some answers might be more useful than others. Alternatively, if you can choose multiple ways to address the
same question – for example, your data source might have both
the number of transfusions and the information necessary to calculate the estimated blood loss with at least one formula – you
might try each approach in turn, either showing that your results
are robust or subject to variation.

EXAMPLE 2: COMORBIDITIES AND MORTALITY

You've probably got some familiarity with the Charlson
Comorbidity Index (CCI), which is used as a way to score how
sick a patient is. Used as a predictor in a model, it can control
what contribution a patient's overall condition makes to outcomes. Details of the CCI's history and implementation are relevant to the purpose of this book.

The original Charlson study [36] pre-dates modern administrative databases. Out of 607 patients admitted to a single medical service in a single month in 1984, the Charlson study had
both hospital charts and one-year follow-up data for 559 patients.
From this population, a Cox proportional hazards model was
used to derive a comorbidity index. The index was then tested on
its ability to predict 10-year survival for 685 women with breast
cancer treated between 1962 and 1969 at a different institution.

The Charlson paper is a classic, and external validation at
another institution is always a good way to support findings,
but the paper does not explain why a breast cancer cohort was
selected in particular. Also, the later widespread use of the CCI
seems ironic given the statement in their discussion that "it cannot be viewed as the final, definitive study because the number of
patients with any given level of serious of a comorbid disease is
relatively small." However, in a later, a larger study based on ICD-
9-CM coding to detect Charlson comorbidities in 27,111 patients,
Deyo et al. [37] showed that the Charlson index was associated
with a variety of health outcomes such as hospital charges, length

of stay, and of course mortality, but the story does not end there. Later, Quan and colleagues added ICD-10-CM coding [38] to extend the model to the new coding system but then derived an updated weighting scheme [39] to account for changes in medical technology since 1984 and found that some comorbidities actually dropped out of the updated CCI.

The lesson here is that even when your findings are generalizable to multiple populations, outcomes, or settings, they may still not be once-and-for-all definitive because future developments can always change things.

EXAMPLE 3: MINIMAL CLINICALLY IMPORTANT DIFFERENCE

A popular way of assessing a patient's situation is the Patient Reported Outcome (PRO) questionnaire. Depending on the domain of the questionnaire, a PRO may measure pain, function, satisfaction, or general quality of life. Designing and validating these PRO tools is another area of statistics, but a specific piece of it is going to be discussed here as an example of how simple concepts can be difficult in practice.

The minimal clinically important difference (MCID), also called the minimally important difference, is the least change in a PRO that can have a meaningful result to a patient. As with the blood loss during surgery, this seems a simple concept. There are at least nine ways of estimating this simple concept [40]. Some methods focus on estimating the smallest change that can be statistically determined from the available data, a version of the MCID that is also called the minimum detectable difference or MDC. Other methods estimate the MCID as the difference in change scores between patients reporting improvement and those reporting no improvement. There is also an approach based on the receiver operating characteristic (ROC) curve, where the ROC curve is used to select the change in PRO score optimally associated with classification into "improved" or "not improved." Further considering that different studies might use different definitions for improvement and that there can be variations between clinical groups such as the type of treatment and the reason for treatment, there can be considerable variations among MCID estimates (reviewed in [41]).

EXAMPLE 4: THE PARTICULAR PROBLEM OF BMI

The BMI seems convenient but of course really is not. Consider that the BMI is based on weight divided by height-squared. Revisiting basic science, the volume has a cubic dimension – height, width, and depth. Then is using height-squared consistent? It could be argued that a person's height is not affected by weight gain, but the other two dimensions are. A counter-argument is, why not use weight divided by height? This doesn't get into how much of the weight is muscle.

Richard Kronmal [42] goes into detail about why BMI is troublesome statistically. He presents a sample case where the outcome is associated with height or with weight but not both, and the BMI alone is not associated. Therefore, using BMI alone would be misleading. Conversely, if BMI was associated with the outcome, it still would not be clear whether it was because the patient was heavier – it could also be because the patient was shorter. He also points out it's a violation of a good statistical practice – if you include an interaction between variables, a good practice is to also include the main effects of the variables. Kronmal's recommendation is that if you include BMI as a predictor, include also weight and $1/\text{height}^2$ as predictors.

Another issue to consider using BMI as a predictor is that unhealthy patients can be underweight. If underweight patients are in your data set, you may want to graph weight or BMI versus the outcome to check whether there's a tendency for both underweight and overweight patients to show an increased risk of poor outcomes. If so, then the curvature should be included in the regression model.

CHAPTER 11

All Things Being Equal – But How? (Designing the Study)

RANDOM ASSIGNMENT IS NOT ALWAYS AN OPTION

A research question might be framed "All things being equal, what's the expected effect of the treatment?" or "Everything else being equal, what's the difference in outcome between patients with these characteristics?" The problem is how to establish the background condition of all other factors being equal.

The gold standard is to assign someone randomly to a treatment or other controllable factor such as what surgical approach to use. If group membership was randomly assigned, and the groups were large enough, we could assume that all other factors were balanced between groups. The beauty of random assignment is that we do not need to list these other factors or know how they affect the outcome. The assumption, and this gets back to the law of large numbers, is that if the groups are large enough, they will have equal distributions of all of the other potential factors of interest. We can apply our statistical tests assuming all things are equal, but may still want to check that assumption for ourselves.

But supposing you were interested in the difference between diabetic and non-diabetic patients. It is neither possible nor ethical to assign someone to diabetes. Ethics can also kick in even for controllable factors. We can assign someone to a treatment, but then there's another ethical issue, known technically as *equipoise*. Random assignment to treatments is only permissible if there is substantial uncertainty which treatment is better for the patient. Similarly, assigning treatment versus no treatment is only allowed if there is a doubt whether the treatment has an effect.

Assigning treatments is only an option with a prospective study when you are recruiting patients specifically for that study and observing them going forward. If you have a collection of data generated by years of patient care, analysis of that dataset will be a retrospective study. Even if you are collecting data prospectively for the benefit of possible future studies, the studies themselves are still retrospective because the data will not have been specifically gathered to address a research question such as "how does assigning this treatment affect outcome?"

Nothing stops us from doing a simple statistical test comparing outcomes between any two treatment groups in a retrospective data set, but the results may be distorted by ignored differences between groups. For example, one treatment might be favored for sicker or older patients. If the simple comparison indicated that this treatment had worse outcomes, is that the effect of treatment or the effect of more fragile patients? And if the comparison indicated the treatment had a weak or negligible effect, might a stronger effect emerge if the other differences between patient groups were accounted for?

If all things are not equal in the first place, how do we make them that way? There is a large body of work on how to do that. We are only going to skim the surface here.

MATCHING AND STRATIFICATION

Two approaches which are practical if only a few factors are being controlled for are matching and stratification. Each is a simple way of forcing all things to be equal. But each becomes impractical if you are comparing more than two groups or controlling for many covariaties.

In *matching*, for each patient in the smaller group, find corresponding patients in the other group who are close matches in measurable factors such as age, gender, body mass index (BMI) or Charlson comorbidity index. Ideally, a paired analysis should be done to reflect the matching. The matching can be automated by telling the computer for each case, select controls with the same (gender, race, presence of a given condition) or close (height, weight, age) covariates. However, this can become tricky if there are a lot of covariates or some rare conditions where matches cannot be found.

In *stratification*, patients are divided into strata based on the factors of interest – say, males < 65, males ≥65, females < 65, females ≥65. Then the analysis is done within between treatment groups within each strata. There is no pairing to be concerned with in the analysis, but now we have smaller sample sizes within each strata and may have to consider adjusting for multiple comparisons because we have multiple strata.

SELECTING MULTIPLE PREDICTORS

Maybe we aren't interested in all things being equal. The patient will arrive in the office with a collection of relevant demographics, symptoms, and other conditions, and so could ask, "Given my specific circumstances, what can you tell me about increased risks I might face?"

Multivariable statistical models have become a common tool for accounting for many extraneous factors. Any statistical software will offer them. You may remember, perhaps not fondly, studying linear algebra which was a way of manipulating several equations at once – and no, we are not going to review linear algebra anywhere in this book, so you can relax. We mention linear algebra only because multivariate models use them to build on the simple "bivariate" analyses with one predictor and one outcome such as regressions or t-tests.

We won't discuss specifics of multivariable model construction and output here, either, as there is too much variation among model types and software packages; however, some general points are worth discussing.

- Each model will return two estimates for a predictor: the estimated size of the effect, and the estimated uncertainty in the size estimate. There are two ways to get a p-value for a model parameter – either from the two uncertainty estimates or from the observed improvement in model performance due to the inclusion of the parameter.

- Controlling for a predictor associated with both treatment and outcome, the technical definition of a confounder gives you a better assessment of the effect of the treatment on outcome. Controlling for a predictor only associated with the outcome can still improve your estimate by removing variation associated with that nuisance predictor. Either way, this assumes that this predictor has an effect on outcome and/or treatment, not the other way around. Controlling for a "predictor" that is actually caused by your treatment and/or your outcome can distort your analysis. Think about what's the cause and what's the effect.

- Predictor effects are assumed to be independent of each other. That is, the effect of the patient being diabetic is the same whether the patient is older or younger, male or female, or so on. Yes, in this case, "independent" is another way to say "all things being equal." Each estimate can be viewed as being adjusted for all other included factors. It is possible to explicitly define *interaction* terms that allow for predictors to interact, for example, a treatment having different effects in males and females. Interaction terms can be annoying to deal with, but they can also be misleading if you do not include them!

• An advantage of the multivariable model with explicitly defined predictors is that it allows the overall prediction (complication rate, length of stay, etc.) to be calculated conditional on the values of the predictors. Although multivariable models force the researcher to explicitly account for "extraneous" factors, it can be useful to demonstrate whether the observed effect of these factors is consistent with existing knowledge and expectations. A multivariable model based on past patients can be used to make an overall prediction for a new patient.

There is a considerable debate [29, 43] over the best way to select predictors. There's a technical point known as the bias-variance trade-off. An example is shown in Figure 11.1. To noisy data, we fit both a straight line and a polynomial. The straight-line throws away the curvature that the polynomial captures – but which is more accurate? Remember the view of probability as a flowing river. We want to describe the river in a way that's valid whenever we step into it.

We discussed in Chapter 7 that statistical tests try to estimate parameters describing how the observed data can be separated into systematic effects and random variation. If we overfit, our model may try to fit the noise as if it were the signal. If we underfit, we have the opposite risk of losing potentially useful findings; we bias our model by oversimplifying it. Overfitting is a consequence of using too many parameters, perhaps using a polynomial where a line would do, and means that what held for your data when you collected it may not hold for another data set collected at a different time, even from the same patient pool at the same institution. But underfitting will also give you wrong predictions. It's basic science that distance is $0.5 \times$ acceleration $\times$ time^2. However, a straight-line regression to time versus distance

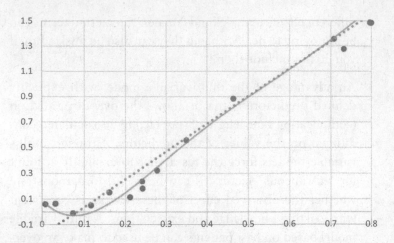

FIGURE 11.1   Example of underfitting versus overfitting. The blue dots are the raw data. The dotted line is a straight-line regression which ignores the apparent curvature at the bottom. The solid line is a polynomial that accounts for the curvature. Which one is more appropriate depends on whether the curvature can be considered a real characteristic of the data or an artifact due to noise.

for constant acceleration will return a result that will be statistically significant and useless at best. An example of underfitting is coming up in Figure 11.2 (Anscombe's quartet, plot II).

What's the best way to pick parameters, given what we don't know about the data? (Famous line: if we knew what we were doing, it wouldn't be research.) Plotting the data for visible trends is always good. So including factors we expect should have an effect, such as age for mortality. But ·what can we do with the statistical tools at hand?

One approach is to use bivariate tests with a looser p-value threshold, say 0.1 or 0.2, to identify values to include. We would want a looser threshold because some predictors may not have a detectable effect unless other predictors are accounted for. An example of this is mortality, where some effects may not be visible until age is accounted for. For that reason, another approach is to start off with a model including all factors and systematically

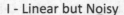

I - Linear but Noisy

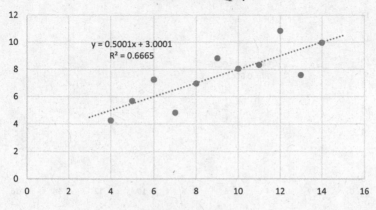

$$y = 0.5001x + 3.0001$$
$$R^2 = 0.6665$$

II- Curved, no noise

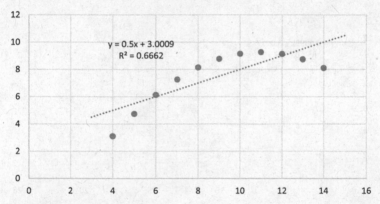

$$y = 0.5x + 3.0009$$
$$R^2 = 0.6662$$

FIGURE 11.2   Anscome's quarter of four different data sets resulting in the same regression line.

prune it of predictors with the least effect on model performance. This is known as backward stepwise regression [29, 43], and we used it in generating predictive scores for operative outcomes [44, 45].

Stepwise regression strategies have drawbacks as the variable selection may be due to chance, but every statistical package offers the tool. Issues can be minimized by using backward selection instead of forward selection, which is adding variables based

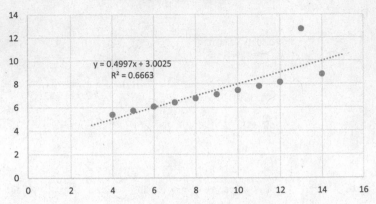

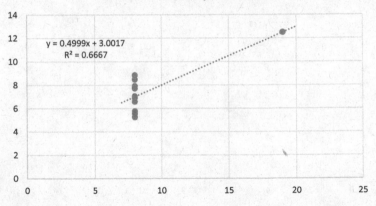

FIGURE 11.2 (Continued)

on the highest impact; using Akaike Information Criterion, a combination of model complexity and model accuracy, to select parameters for removal; and using as much data as possible [46]. We can also use penalized logistic regression [29], where the penalty is applied to the number and size of the regression coefficients, forcing a more conservative model, and bootstrap validation [29, 43] where the model is tested against multiple randomized samples of the data. Frank Harrell [29] provides two pieces of advice for dealing with interaction terms. First, you can do a quick comparison of a model without any interactions to a model with all potential interactions of interest and see if the interaction model gets you any real gain in predictive power; if not, don't worry about interactions. If you are keeping interactions in a model you are pruning systematically, prune interaction terms before pruning main effects. Of course, if your study is motivated by testing for the presence of a particular predictor or interaction, you may want to keep it in as you prune other parameters and keep it in your final model. It is possible you may be presented with a trade-off between models where keeping an interaction term produces a slight but real improvement in model accuracy but costs intuitive clarity. Our recommendation is that if space permits, present both models, or as Yogi Berra reportedly said, "When you see a fork in the road – take it!".

It is important to never let the algorithm do all the thinking. Even if there is a choice of two models and one seems to have better statistical properties, if a model is completely inconsistent with common sense or clinical judgment, it should not be accepted blindly. It should not be rejected automatically, either; if a nonsensical model returns good results, then you should give some thought as to why. In published studies using an administrative database to predict in-hospital mortality [47, 48], some comorbidities such as obesity and depression were listed as being protective – patients with these conditions listed had less chance of dying in hospital. A suggested explanation [47] is that patients who had many serious conditions were less likely to have relatively minor conditions coded, while relatively healthy patients were likelier to have such conditions coded if observed. This explanation does not consider the additional possibility that some patients are at higher risk of dying prior to hospital admission, and so might not be included in the analysis cohorts.

Any predictor selection method should be guided by clinical knowledge of what factors are expected to affect the outcome or those factors that are unknown but of immediate interest. Computational methods should never be seen as a substitute for clinical insight or for thinking through the mechanisms by which a predictor might affect the outcome. No statistical model, no matter how sophisticated, can be expected to account for variables that are absent from the data altogether. Assuming too simple of a model can throw out important information. A model with too many parameters may be fit to statistical noise as well as to real effects, and so appear too optimistic.

Further, if two predictors are correlated with each other, then the model may not be able to detect whether either one of them is actually associated with the outcome, and neither one may appear to be useful. This phenomenon is called *collinearity*, and those readers fondly remembering linear algebra may be thinking of the consequences of a set of equations being of less than full rank. Having collinear predictors won't ruin a model's ability to predict outcomes, but it will mean that model coefficients will be nonsensical. We remember one study where predictors were highly correlated, and we had to discuss with the researcher which measurements should be retained. In this case, criteria for keeping predictors included which measurements were noisier than others and which measurements were likelier to be used by other clinicians. You can check for collinearity by any of the following: (a) test statistically for correlations between predictors; (b) systematically add and remove predictors and see if other predictor values change; or (c) use a "variance inflation factor" which some statistical packages can return and which will tell you which parameters are potentially affected by correlations with other parameters.

Of course, if you have a polynomial, you expect some relationship between x and x^2. If you are concerned about that adding to collinearity, you could create a new variable $x_0 = x - \text{mean}(x)$, and use x_0 and x_0^2 in your statistical model. Subtracting the mean will remove much of the correlation between polynomial terms.

The prediction of a model can be seen as the conditional mean of the outcome – remember conditional probability? – given that the predictors have a certain set of values. That is, the predicted outcome is the expected value (mean) of the distribution of outcome values, conditional on the values of the predictors. The residual is the difference between the actual outcome and this conditional mean, and the regression model typically assumes that residuals follow a Gaussian distribution with 0 mean. That is, the measurement error is purely random. In practice, the residual is going to be a combination of random variation and structural issues in the model: real data is not obliged to follow a convenient mathematical formula. (Also note that this discussion of residuals is not relevant for a logistic regression which is based on a binary outcome.)

The statistical equivalent of an x-ray for regressions is to plot residuals on the y-axis and the model prediction on the x-axis. The regression assumptions predict that the plot will be flat and have equal variation at all points along the x-axis. If the spread of residuals is different for low predictions than for high predictions, then you have a skewed distribution (as discussed in Chapter 4) and that a linear model with outcome as-is may not be appropriate; approaches are considered in Chapter 9.

The residual plot may also show that the model is wrong, whether or not the regression assumptions are correct. If the residuals aren't flat, then you may need to add another predictor, as there may be variation not accounted for in the model. There may also be an interaction, where the patient's demographic or clinical factors can affect how well the patient responds to treatment; for example, how smoking can affect wound healing after surgery.

Figure 11.2 shows four examples, known as Anscombe's quartet, of how an outcome can depend on a predictor. In these four cases, the regression line and correlation coefficient are identical even though the relationships are clearly different. We should reiterate here that the regression and correlation coefficient, as calculated by textbook or Excel, are only meaningful in the first case. The correlation coefficient will still describe the proportion of observed variation in Y that can be explained by X subject to the assumptions made in a regression – but only the first case in Figure 11.2 is consistent with those assumptions.

You'll see Anscombe's quartet in a number of places, including Wikipedia, but here we're taking it one slight step further (Figure 11.3) to show how residuals – the differences between the regression predictions and the actual values – can be used to check a regression. For case I, where the assumptions of regression are met, we see the ideal case for residual versus predicted – a flat line with no

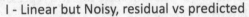

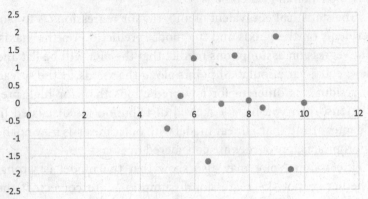

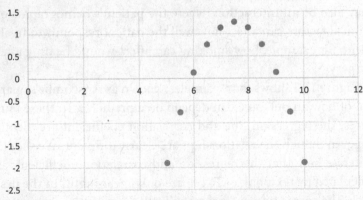

FIGURE 11.3   Residuals for two cases in Anscombe's quartet.

systematic pattern. For case II, where the straight line was fit to visibly curved data, we see a pattern in the residuals. When you do a diagnostic plot like this, it is important to plot the residuals against *predicted* (fitted) values, not the actual observed values. The math behind the regression means that the residuals should not be correlated with the predictions but will be correlated with the observations. Showing that the residual is associated with the observations doesn't tell you anything. It's when you see a pattern in residual versus fitted values you know there may be an issue.

PROPENSITY SCORES

An alternative approach to handling multiple predictors is to generate *propensity scores*, which estimate the probability of the patient being in a particular group based on the data available. Logistic regression or another method is used to estimate the probability of patients being assigned to a treatment given other predictors that could also affect the outcome. Unlike logistic regression for analysis, we are not interested in pruning parameters: we want the full range of predictors that are expected to affect the outcome. These probability estimates are the propensity scores, and they can be used in a number of ways.

1) Weigh the patients going into a simple bivariate comparison. The propensity score weighting should effectively balance the distribution of factors between groups as if the groups were randomized in the first place, and this assumption can be examined by using tables of weighted variable distributions.

2) Stratification or matching, as before. We would not use a paired analysis here because two patients may have the same propensity score but based on different variables. Also, Gary King [49] points out that the matching is often done based on random draws from the data set so the results may

vary considerably. Propensity score stratification would not have these issues.

3) Propensity scores can be used as predictors themselves, substituting for the predictors that went into the propensity score. This can be useful if there are a large number of predictors for the data. However, for large data sets, this may not be useful.

However propensity scores are used, they should be compared between patients based on the group membership being predicted. You want to confirm that the propensity scores overlap between groups. If they do not, then using propensity scores in any of the ways above may have problems. Another imitation of propensity scores cannot balance predictors that were not recorded in the first place.

ALSO CONSIDER

No matter how many predictors you use, in a plot, you are practically limited to a main predictor and perhaps a grouping variable that controls line color, thickness, etc. Depending on the situation, you may also be able to add another variable for subplots of data subgroups. However, such plots can still be informative and can add another perspective on the analysis results. Also, it may still be worth doing a simple X versus Y analysis to see how an outcome depends on a single predictor of interest, and whether that relationship varies when other parameters are included.

Comparisons should be unambiguous. For example, consider two groups of patients, one seen by surgeon A who always uses method B, and one seen by surgeon C who always uses method D. Perhaps we've randomized patients to surgeons A and C, and perhaps this is a retrospective study. Either way, we will never be able to distinguish, in this situation, differences between surgeons A and C and differences between methods B and D. What we can do is find as many surgeons as we can who use either method (and we may even find a few who use both!) and include all their patients in the data set. Then statistical analyses methods can separate the variation due to surgeons from the variation due to method. We might even be able to make a statement about whether differences between methods have a greater impact than differences between surgeons.

Also, remember that not all data records may themselves be equal. Suppose the outcome of interest is the average blood glucose measurement during a hospital stay. Some patients may have more measurements than others, so their estimated averages should be relatively more reliable. One way to account for this is to weight data so that the records based on more measurements have a higher weight. Another approach is to use mixed models, as described in Chapter 13.

There is a body of work on the topic of *causal inference*, which is concerned with the question of potential outcomes. In the real world, the patient either gets operated on or doesn't. We can observe the outcome for patients who received a treatment but can only estimate what it would have been for the same patients if they did not get the treatment, and similarly we can observe the outcome for patients who were not treated but can only estimate what it would have been if they were treated. Estimates of the unobserved outcomes are plugged in to create estimates of the casual effect of treatment. Tools used include *difference-in-difference* methods, which use interaction terms in a regression to estimate before-and-after effects given that the patient did receive treatment, and propensity scores to balance treated and untreated groups.

CHAPTER 12

Binary and Count Outcomes

LOGISTIC REGRESSION IS A familiar tool in the medical literature, but how well do you understand it? A binary outcome is constrained to two values, which we can view as 0 or 1. (At the computer level, yes/no, dead/alive, etc. are all mapped to 0/1.) The probability of the outcome being 1 is estimated from the mean of this 0/1 variable and is in turn constrained to be no less than 0 (never happens) and no more than 1 (always happens). But regression equations don't have these constraints.

The trick is to map the interval 0 to 1 (including all percentages) to a wider range of numbers. This is done using the logistic function: $y = 1/(1 + e^{-x})$, where **e** is a very special value in mathematics, about 2.718 (plus a lot of digits we're dropping because otherwise it would go on forever). What makes **e** special is calculus: the derivative of e^x is e^x. This is not a typo but a useful convenience. The derivative of the logistic function can be shown to be $y' = y(1 - y)$, so this simplifies a lot of computational operations that go on behind the scenes. (If you want to set up something to be done with minimal effort, find a math or computer geek. Many are lazy sods just like Dr. Maltenfort.) The important math here is that a logistic regression algorithm estimates the regression equation between a defined set of predictors and the logarithm of p/(1 − p).

Immediately we have a math problem which crops up whenever your logistic regression software cautions you that probabilities of 0 or 1 have emerged. The odds p/(1 − p) are undefined if p is 1. However, the logarithm of the odds is also undefined if the odds are 0 which happens if p equals 0. Your software won't crash but observe your results carefully.

Logistic regression is an example of what's called a generalized linear model (GLM). One difference between GLMs and linear regression is that linear regression can be calculated in one pass using linear algebra methods, while a GLM has to be solved iteratively, with an initial estimate being improved over multiple passes. While a linear regression requires a Gaussian distribution of residuals, which is the difference between expected and observed values, generalized linear models can use a range of distributions. This is useful for dealing with count data.

If a binary variable can take the value 0 or 1, count data can be seen as the combination of a series of binary events – for example, a patient might have a certain probability of being discharged on any given day (a yes or no event), but until the discharge length of stay accumulates. Costs can accumulate similarly. Such count data will often have a skewed distribution – many smaller values and few larger ones.

Count data is usually assumed to follow a Poisson or a negative binomial distribution. Both of these are related to the binomial distribution, which describes the probability of different observation counts given a probability and a certain number of trials. The Poisson distribution describes the probability of seeing so many events in a given interval. It assumes that the variance of the outcome will increase with the mean value of the outcome, which is an important distinction from linear regression, which assumes all values are equally noisy regardless of size. However, it also assumes the variance equals the mean, which can be an issue if there is extra variation in the data.

If we use Poisson regression (a GLM based on the Poisson distribution), we have to check for *overdispersion*, which is when the data has variation the Poisson distribution doesn't account for and which can introduce extra uncertainty in regression estimates. Software that allows for Poisson regression usually allows for both checking and adjusting for overdispersion. Alternatively, you can use negative binomial regression (if available). The negative binomial distribution describes the probability of seeing a given number of non-events before a total number of events are observed. The negative binomial is a bit more complicated because the computer has to estimate two parameters instead of one but does not have to worry about overdispersion. There is such a thing as *underdispersion* when the data shows less variability than expected, but the consequence of underdispersion is that our margins of error may be unduly pessimistic, which is of less concern than false optimism. Note that overdispersion and underdispersion will not affect the actual parameter estimates in the regression, just the amount of uncertainty estimated for them.

One issue that comes up with GLMs is that sometimes the coefficients aren't in the most useful form. For example, logistic regression returns odds ratios. The risk ratio is intuitive: just the ratio between probabilities. However, what does that mean if the reference probability is 0.8 and the risk ratio is 1.5? A probability of 1.2 does not make sense as probabilities have to be between 0 and 1 – nothing can have more than a 100% chance of happening, or less than a 0% chance. Odds ratios are more flexible. Similarly, Poisson and negative binomial regression return parameters that correspond to percentage increases. A patient with a particular condition may have a 15% longer length of stay than a patient without, but putting that in context requires knowing what the expected length of stay without would be. We will discuss how to present various types of statistical result in Chapter 15, but the general advice we would give you is to use the regression model to generate predictions for cases of interest (for example, a

45-year-old patient with general versus localized anesthesia) and see how they compare.

This is just glossing over GLMs. For example, binary data can also be treated with probit and complementary log-log models, which make slightly different statistical assumptions than the logistic model but whose parameters are much less intuitive. Generalized additive models are a variation of GLM and allow for more complicated effects of predictors, but the trade-off is that the models can be harder to interpret. There is also a nice parlor trick with GLMs where you use what is called an "identity link" instead of the transformation usually associated with the GLM. The downsides are that the analysis might crash because of unrealistic numbers (such as negatives for count data) and that your statistical model might not be as good a fit as the model with the preferred (technical name: *canonical*) transformation, but if it works the parameters will be additive terms on the scale of the outcome; for example, you could get additive risk instead of an odds ratio.

CHAPTER 13

Repeated Measurements and Accounting for Change

S UPPOSE A PATIENT DOES not ask, "Where will I be after surgery?" but "how much will I improve after surgery?" These are not exactly the same questions. Think of a patient with a pain score measured on a 0–10-point scale. You may not be able to say, "After surgery, your pain will be 2 out of 10, no worse." You could say something like, "Based on studies, the average patient sees a 1.5 point drop in pain." However, that's going to mean something different to patients who have different pre-operative pain levels. A patient with a baseline pain score of 2 would expect to be almost pain-free. A patient with a baseline pain score of 8 may not consider 1.5 points enough improvement to return to normal functioning.

If we have data collected on a group of patients at the beginning of treatment and at the end of treatment, we can test whether they improved after treatment. If we have another group of patients who did not get the treatment but were measured at the same time in the same place, we can estimate the potential effect of treatment. However, once we begin looking at the same patient on multiple occasions, we have a new issue to consider. Statistical tests assume all observations are independent. A study with repeated observations violates this assumption so these tests become inappropriate. The technical name for this is *pseudoreplication*, and it can be addressed properly, if you use statistical tests that account for multiple measurements from the same source.

To illustrate pseudoreplication, consider a study with 100 subjects, each observed at the same five times. How much data do we have? We have more data than if we had simply observed 100 subjects at a single time. However, we don't have as much data as if we had observed 500 individual people because observations coming from the same person are presumably correlated with each other.

Comparing paired and unpaired t-tests can further illustrate this point. Unpaired t-tests are when there is no relationship between individual members across the two groups being compared. Paired t-tests are when a relationship exists. The most relevant example here would be clinical scores for the same individual at different times, such as before and after treatment. The paired t-test is actually an unpaired t-test; the quantity being tested is the difference between the patient's before and after scores, and the comparison is against a constant value of 0. The patient's score at a given time can be assumed to be the sum of three parts: the treatment effect, random variation, and a constant part that is intrinsic to the patient. By taking the difference, we are left with the treatment effect and random variation – the constant part, present both before and after, is subtracted out. We didn't even have to estimate it; as in a randomized study, it cancelled out.

Of course, it's not that simple in the long run. There's a well-known statistical paradox, called Lord's Paradox, which was discovered in a study of the effects of the college diet in males and females. The data was analyzed in two ways. One approach was to take the net change in weight, the difference between before and after scores, and see if that was different between men and women. The other way was to use a statistical model predicting the final weight from the initial weight and the gender. The paradox, of course, is that the two methods made different implications about whether sex affected the final weight. The resolution to the paradox is that the two approaches ask different questions. Method (1) is a t-test and Method (2) is a regression line. As mathematical statements:

Method (1): (Final − Initial) = $GenderEffect_1$ + e

Method (2): Final = m * Initial + $GenderEffect_2$ + e

The difference between the two approaches is that the first method forces the slope m to be 1.0. The second method allows m to be calculated by the regression in order to minimize the estimated value of the random error term e. For simplicity, we're not showing constant or intercept terms, but, again, Method 1 would force the intercept to be 0, while Method 2 would allow it to vary and might have more statistical power due to the greater flexibility. The take-home message here is that the results of an analysis are dependent on the assumptions made in the analysis and that these assumptions can be implicit in the methods applied. For a thorough review, see Judea Pearl's article "Lord's Paradox Revisited – (Oh Lord! Kumbaya!)" [50].

This is just for two points in time. What about three or more? Or situations where the patients are each measured at different times? Also consider that in the same way, a regression might have time or distance as a predictor, a single study may follow the same group of patients across time or may ask the same question of patients at different sites. From the level of computation, these are similar questions.

Of course, a study can be both longitudinal and multi-site. While it seems like a reach to throw meta-analyses into the mix, a meta-analysis can be viewed as a multi-site study scattered in time. The meta-analysis may not have detailed per-patient information and may be based on prospective and retrospective studies, but the specific math used to account for variations per study site is very similar.

A popular but inefficient approach for longitudinal data is to apply a separate statistical test to compare patient groups at each time point. Not only does this throw out information about the patient at other time points, but it means that you have as many p-values and estimated differences as you have time points. Another inefficient approach for multiple measurements is to average measurements taken in the same time frame per patient, as this throws out important information about the variability of the data.

A better approach is to use a *mixed-effects* model that can account for repeated measurements from the same person and for patients grouped by what site they were observed at. A strength of mixed-effects models is that you can account for multiple grouping factors in the same model and that the estimated contribution of each of these factors can be informative. These grouping factors are called *random effects* to distinguish them from *fixed effects*. In an ordinary regression, all predictors are fixed effects. Think of them as having a fixed frame of reference (age, gender, etc.).

In one sense, the random effect is itself a categorical variable, with parameters assigned to each random effect level. The difference is in how it's calculated. For fixed effects, a categorical variable with N levels will have N − 1 parameters associated with it, with one value taken as a reference level. For random effects with N levels, there will be N parameters that are presumed to arise from a Gaussian distribution with a mean of 0. A model without random effects will try to estimate the components of variation due to systematic effects and randomness. The model with random effects will also estimate a third component of variation among individuals.

Looking back at the inefficient approach of one test per time point, you would be faced with one test result per time point.

However, the mixed model allows you to make an overall statement about whether the treatment has an effect and whether the treatment effect is dependent on time – perhaps the treatment effect takes a while to kick in or perhaps the benefit of the treatment is only short-term. There are still parameter estimates and standard errors at each time point so you can examine the trajectory of the outcome.

Another advantage of the mixed-effects model is that it does not require that each patient have a measurement at each time point. If patients miss a visit or drop out of the study, the information they provide at other time points still informs the overall model.

However, the "Lord's Paradox" question is still there – do you want to include baseline measurements as a predictor or as an outcome? Leaving baseline as an outcome may be more intuitive – you can say whether two treatment groups have statistically different values at baseline, and the outcome parameters compare each time point to baseline. On the other hand, you may have more statistical power using baseline value as a predictor. As with other topics, analyzing changes from baseline is not trivial; for example, if a patient has a more extreme initial situation (say, high pain or low function score), then they have the possibility of a greater change as they approach normal; a patient with a less extreme start isn't about to change by the same magnitude if that would mean they became better than normal. The problems with change scores have been assessed in detail in posts by Frank Harrell [51, 52], who opined elsewhere that there's a difference between forecasting the amount of rain and deciding whether to take an umbrella; the related point is that the net amount of improvement, the difference between baseline and final, may not be as relevant to the patient as the actual final score.

Information comes out of the model in terms of the potential contribution of each specific level and the variance of the associated distribution. The *intraclass correlation coefficient* is the fraction of variation in the outcome that can be attributed to the random effect; if the residual error is small compared to the random effect, the intraclass correlation coefficient will approach 1.0.

In the same way that a generalized linear model (logistic or Poisson regression) is an extension of linear regression, the generalized linear mixed model (GLMM) is an extension of the linear mixed model. GLMM coefficients can be interpreted comparably – that is, you can get an odds ratio from a fixed-effects or mixed-effects logistic regression. However, interpreting the relative size of random effect variance and total variance may be trickier. The prediction from a mixed-effects or GLMM model may be made specific to the level of the random effects or may neglect the random effect contribution altogether to estimate expected values for individuals.

There are other tools available such as generalized estimating equations or conditional logistic regression, but they do not allow for multiple factors and do not give the same information estimates. If you are at the point where you are choosing between these approaches, you are beyond the scope of the book and should be consulting with a statistician.

CHAPTER 14

What If the Data
Is Not All There?

NOT ALL MISSING DATA is missing in the same way. There are a number of reasons why data may be unavailable. The data may not have been recorded in the first place. Review for outliers may have detected and thrown out improperly recorded or otherwise suspicious data. Whatever the cause, the result is holes in the dataset – outcomes without predictors or predictors without outcomes.

There are three technical labels for these holes. *Missing completely at random* (MCAR) is when the data is lost because of chance effects that have nothing to do with predictors or outcomes. For example, a lab value might be missing because the testing equipment was not available that day. MCAR is the best situation; you can analyze complete data with no risk of bias, just some loss of precision. *Missing at random* (MAR) is when the chance of missing data is associated with the observed data. For example, in a multi-center study, one center may have lab equipment that is less reliable. Both MCAR and MAR can be addressed by statistical tools. *Missing not at random* (MNAR) is the problem case where the data is associated with unobservable parameters; perhaps a site simply doesn't report a particular lab, or patients with more extreme lab values aren't available for the study in the first place or are likelier to drop out of the study.

The preferred practice for MAR or MCAR is something called *multiple imputation*. "Imputation" is just a fancy word for "filling in the blank." Multiple imputation generates multiple plausible replacement values, which can each be used in an analysis and then the results are combined. The imputation algorithm bases the replacements on observable relationships among the data, which is why it does not work for MNAR. The analysis of MNAR data will have to be designed with consideration for why the data is missing.

Multiple imputation is preferable to single imputation because it accounts for potential variability in the replacement. Single imputation runs the risk of biasing the results. For example, if you replace a missing continuous value with its overall mean, then you have a value that does not reflect the relationships between variables in the dataset, nor does it include the random error that affects other measurements. This is also a problem with "last observation carried forward" in longitudinal studies.

Multiple imputation methods usually give two options for generating replacements. One is called *predictive mean matching*, and it finds suitable values in the existing data that can fill in the blank. This is useful that the new values will have a comparable range – you won't see an age filled in with a negative number, for example. The alternative is to use regression to generate a new value. This may not be in the existing range, but that may be what you want. For example, it is common to get back lab results with a "<x" (where x is a number), showing that the result was lower than some threshold of detectability. A regression imputation may be able to estimate what that measurement would have been by extrapolating from the existing data.

A potential approach for binary data is to compare per variable what would happen if either all missing data was all the one value versus what would happen if all missing data was all the other value. You know the true situation has to be between the two extremes.

If you're in a situation where missing data is a factor, it's worth exploring on your own to assess the situation. For example, it may be informative that a particular group is at higher risk for missing data. Also, consider whether missingness is itself an important factor in your research question. In survey questions, some responses may be blank because they are not applicable to the responder. For a predictive model based on admissions or claims data, it can be meaningful to use "missing" data as a level of a predictive categorical variable.

A particular missing data situation can occur in a randomized study, where patients who receive a particular treatment arm may drop out. Perhaps they were not compliant; perhaps they transferred to another treatment. In this particular case, you want to run your statistical model as if the patients were in the arm they were assigned to. This is called an *intention to treat analysis* and allows you to test the results of the policy of assigning a patient to treatment [53]. Although this would arguably bias results in indicating no effect between treatments, that result may be what you want if the study was intended to show potential benefits of a new treatment. If you are designing a study, you should include not only the potential use of an intention to treat analysis but also ways of ensuring that you continue to receive data from patients who discontinue or switch treatments.

There is no statistical tool for accounting for what you don't know, especially if you don't know that you don't know it. A database may list a diagnosis but not the lab values or observations leading up to the diagnosis, and it will not include diagnoses that have not been made. The patients in a medical practice will always be a biased sample – they chose to work with that clinician. Follow-up data on complications might not be available if the complication was treated at another hospital. The best you can do in those cases is try analyses based on subgroups that you expect to be more homogeneous or less prone to error, for example, patients seen more regularly at the practice.

The importance of missing data may be brought home by the story of the airplanes that returned from combat missions during World War 2. According to the story, a study was done of where the planes showed the most bullet holes. The most holes were seen in wings and fuselage so the plan was to armor the planes at those sites. But a statistician, Abraham Wald, if you want to look the story up, pointed out that the place to armor the planes was at the engine, which showed the least bullet holes. As Wald pointed out, aircraft shot in the engine were the ones least likely to return from the mission.

CHAPTER 15

Showing the Data to Others – Graphs and Tables, Part 2

ORGANIZING THE PRESENTATION

One general rule for preparing the final manuscript is that all the plots and tables should come from the same data pool. This would seem obvious, but our experience has been that over time data files can be revised and requests for analyses can be revised or repeated. The result is often a Frankenstein situation where the pieces of the paper come from different bodies of data.

We distinguish here between papers where the pieces of the paper are from different versions of what should be the same data, resulting in an incoherent story, and papers where different data sources are carefully linked (such as EHR data and Census data) to create a detailed, consistent story.

Whatever your motivation for writing the paper, your goal should be a clear and credible story. You are writing non-fiction (we hope!), but there is still a narrative. Each graph or table should offer a clear piece of the plot, ordered in a way that one idea logically points to the next. The manuscript ties the ideas together and elaborates upon them.

There are unavoidable constraints. You can only fit so many plots on a page, so a 4×4 grid of subplots is probably impractical. Journals will probably have limits of how many graphs or tables you can have, and often a journal presented with plots labelled 1A, 1B, and 1C will count them as three separate plots. Also, will you be expecting the graph to be viewed on-screen or printed? Printed documents are likely to be in black and white, so your colors will be lost. On the other hand, some viewers of a web page or live presentation may be color-blind so you should consider the palette you are using.

The manuscript, including tables and plots, is an instrument for telling the story. Make your decisions based on how best to tell the story to your intended audience. Part of the process will be ensuring that the pieces are kept in context that your reader will understand immediately. Similarly, you want to present statistical test results in as intuitive a way as possible.

PRESENTING THE NARRATIVE

Abelson's book *Statistics as a Principled Argument* [2] is written from the perspective of how to present an analysis as a set of clear, linked, and convincing statements that put forth the conclusions of the study.

Dr. Abelson offers a MAGIC formula – no, that's not a typo – for what should go into the presentation of results.

Magnitude	How large is the effect
Articulation	Is the story clear?
Generality	How widely does it apply?
Interestingness	What makes this work novel?
Credibility	Are there any flaws in the data or the analysis?

We don't need to elaborate on magnitude here, and articulation is discussed elsewhere in this chapter. Generality refers to how transportable those results are. Say you have data from a large metropolitan hospital; will the findings present any benefits to clinicians working in a small rural area? At the time of writing, questions of income and ethnic disparity are forefront in the news. Your patient mix may also be skewed by comorbidities, either due to local prevalence in your area or because the study design excluded patients with certain comorbid conditions. If any groups have been excluded from your study based on the availability of data or selection criteria (such as being under 18 or being pregnant), the conclusions may not be applicable to them.

Interestingness is of course whether your result is novel. Reading a published study, you may realize you could do the same thing with the data you have at your institution. But should you do the exact same thing? Read that study critically and ask what you would have done differently or what could have been done better. Can you show more precise estimates, a broader population, alternative explanations, or exceptions to the prior study's conclusions? A reviewer at a journal may reject your article on the grounds it's been seen before, and there's nothing new. Of course, this neglects the real and delightful possibility you may be working on something no one has seen or thought of before! More power to you, just be sure to do the statistics right!

Credible, like interesting, will often come up between you and the reviewer when you submit the manuscript. Are you interpreting the analysis correctly? Did you do the right analysis? Is there some limitation in the data that might have impacted your analysis?

KEEPING NUMBERS IN CONTEXT

Jane E. Miller [54], in a paper that can be found online, gives examples of how to improve descriptions of statistical tests in the text. Following her lead, rather than say "age and outcome are correlated (p < 0.01)" or "the regression coefficient between outcome and age is 0.03"; perhaps try "for each year of age, the risk of outcome increases by 3%." If you have multiple regression coefficients, for example, the effect of treatment and the effect of age, consider whether you can put the effect of treatment in the context of how many years of age it corresponds to.

Dr. Miller also recommends changing the scale of units where appropriate for clarity; for example, a study of operative time may have data per minute, but the results may be more intuitive if you can express them per hour or per quarter-hour. John Allen Paulos [55] points out that a dollar a week seems like a very small number, and 15.6 billion dollars a year seems very large. But if you assume 300 million Americans each paying a dollar a week for 52 weeks, you get 15.6 billion.

Scale can also affect the relevance of the number to the audience. For example, a surgeon may perform 500 surgeries of a particular type per year, and let's assume a 1% complication rate. Such surgeons would see five complications a year. A health care organization such as a hospital may have 10–20 such surgeons, and an insurance company will be funding many such hospitals. At this aggregate level, each participant has a motivation in keeping the complication rate as low as possible, and a predictor with an odds ratio of 2 or 3 is of great interest. On the other hand, a patient who only expects to get the surgery once might be very reluctant to change habits, seeing not much difference between a 1% risk and a 3% risk.

It is tempting to be a completist and show everything. However, everything you show is going to be something your reader may want to have explained to them. For example, the intercept is the expected value (or rate) of the outcome at some theoretical baseline. If the goal of your study is to show how patient or clinical factors affect the outcome, then the intercept's main value may be to provide a reference point. For example, a treatment may add six months to life expectancy – but what was the life expectancy before treatment, one month or ten years? Also, if the age or weight are predictors as numerical values, then the intercept describes the expected outcome when these values are zero – which is nonsensical in the real world. You could, in fact, run a regression with a more meaningful intercept by subtracting means out of your continuous predictors then running the regression; the resulting intercept would represent expected outcome at an average age, weight, etc.

Regression coefficients of course get more complicated when you have interaction terms. If your regression shows a treatment by age interaction, for example, then the output will include the main effects of treatment and the age and the interaction term, each with a standard error or confidence interval. Here's a made-up example: we generated data for a thousand cases with ages 30–80 and 50% chance of treatment and then the outcome was 25 * Age + (200 − 5 * Age) If treated + 500 times a Gaussian random variable with mean 0 and SD 1. The linear regression coefficients are:

	Coefficient	Standard error
Intercept	−42.3	89.5
Age effect per year	25.7	1.6
Treatment (yes versus no)	282.9	121.3
Treatment × Age (per year)	−6.3	2.1

with an R-squared of 0.31. Although the noise distorts the treatment variables, note that 282.9/6.3 = 44.9. Without the noise, the treatment by age interaction would cancel out the treatment effect at 200/5 = 40. In the paper, you could put the interaction effect in context by saying something like "the effect of the treatment reverses as age 44.9 (282.9/6.3), decreasing with age." You can also sum the age and treatment by age interaction to say that "with treatment, outcome increases 19.4 (25.7-6.3) per year," or sum up the regression coefficients to get the total effect for the parameters and present a nice table:

Age	Without treatment	With treatment
40	−42.3 + 40 × 25.7 = 985.7	1,028 + 282.9 − 6.3 * 40 = 1,016.6
50	−42.3 + 50 × 25.7 = 1,242.7	1,285 + 282.9 − 6.3 * 50 = 1,210.6
60	−42.3 + 60 × 25.7 = 1,499.7	1,542 + 282.9 − 6.3 * 60 =1,404.6

This is a made-up problem – we generated random ages and treatment and added noise – and you won't be putting the math in the table, just the results. If you're using GLMs such as logistic or Poisson regression, remember to sum the raw coefficients and not the odds ratios etc.

One thing missing from these approaches is an estimate of uncertainty. There are ways to combine the standard errors as you add the coefficients, but unless the original regression was very time-consuming the easiest approach is to re-run the analysis changing the reference from "no treatment" to "treatment." None of the other coefficients will be affected except those involving treatment. For our toy problem, we find that the coefficient for age using Treated as a reference is 19.4 (as expected) with a standard error of 1.4. Also, most statistical software should allow you to make predictions from a model, including standard error – so we have

| Age | Without treatment | | With treatment | |
	Outcome	Standard error	Outcome	Standard error
40	985.7	32.5	1,016.6	29.9
50	1,242.7	23.9	1,210.6	22.0
60	1,499.7	24.1	1,404.6	22.1

TABLES VERSUS GRAPHS: SCALE AND STYLE

Putting results in tables or graphs is as much a matter of personal preference as how the plots or tables are themselves laid out. To some extent, the design of individual plots and tables will be constrained by the requirements of a journal. Dr. Maltenfort and some colleagues once submitted a paper with one figure that had parts A–C, and the journal responded that it considered each part a figure so we had too many figures by their reckoning.

The scale of numbers may be an advantage to the table or the graph, depending on the situation. The size of the numbers in a table is the size of the font. In a graph, the visible difference between numbers is the point – or the line or the bar. If I have two numbers, one very large and one very small, that I want to show in context to each other, the best way to do it may depend on the overall story I am trying to tell.

ARTICULATING THE STORY

When Dr. Maltenfort was in graduate school, his long-suffering mentors kept stressing to him the importance of telling a story. This confused Dr. Maltenfort, which even now is never difficult. Stories had plots and characters and settings. Data was numbers, and the analysis was math. There was an overlap?

The parallel Dr. Maltenfort was missing (then and now, he loses his glasses when they're on top of his head) was that a story begins with a status quo and then through a clear and logically connected series of events, without gaps or confusion or unnecessary digression, arrives at a conclusion where as many loose ends as possible are tied up.

There is no overall approach to telling any narrative. George Orwell, in his 1946 essay "Politics and the English Language," lists six rules for clear writing. Rule 6 was "Break any of these rules sooner than say anything outright barbarous." For us, barbarous would be anything misleading or confusing. Much like the bias-variance tradeoff in multivariable models, sometimes we have to choose between a simpler statement that omits fine details and a detailed statement that risks losing the reader

Dr. Miller offers a potential useful formula in both of her books on writing about statistics [56, 57]: **GEE**. First, make a General statement, and then give a representative Example, finally discuss Exceptions. Following her formula, we might write something like, "We found that the average cost increased approximately 5% per year. A treatment that cost $10,000 in 2005 cost $15,513 in 2015. However, patients discharged to rehab incurred an additional $2,000 in costs."

Dr. Abelson, besides his MAGIC formula, also parses the potential statements that could be made about a study into three types: ticks, buts and blobs. Ticks are positive statements (such as Dr. Miller's general statement and examples), while buts are statements that limit, constrain or modify ticks (such as Dr. Miller's exceptions). Blobs are statements that are factual but are not necessarily meaningful in themselves (such as p-values). He also distinguishes between a "brash" style of presentation which is focused on making the findings sound as good as possible and a "stuffy" style which applies all statistical rules strictly, and recommends a balance between the two to maintain the advantages of speculating about and exploring data and of maintaining reasonable caution in interpreting results.

VISUAL LINGO

There is a wealth of excellent texts on how to present graphs, charts, plots, etc., including how to organize and highlight tables to better lead the reader through it. Along with Dr. Miller's books, we also recommend Edward Tufte's *The Visual Display of Quantitative Information* [58] as one of the definitive texts on how to create graphs with high information and minimal clutter. A more recent book, Cole Nussbaumer Knaflic's *Storytelling with Data* [59], shows a variety of ways to improve communication using charts and tables.

Not even we would try to consolidate all of that information here, but we will share a few high points based on our own reading and experience. This is based largely on what we find to be visual expectations on the part of the audience. How you approach such expectations is of course a matter of individual preference, but ignoring them risks losing the reader's attention or comprehension.

A line going left to right implies a trend as some quantity is increasing. This might be the calendar year, age, or BMI. A scatterplot shows the variation in the data but not average values. If you show the average, either by calculating the mean for a category or plotting a regression line, you may still have to indicate the variation. We say "may" because sometimes error bars or shaded confidence intervals need to be dropped to make the figure clearer. What actually goes into a figure should be those minimal details absolutely necessary to tell the story adequately. Anything more is clutter.

Although the bar plot with error bars is common, the boxplot discussed in Chapter 6 is more informative. You can emphasize a trend by drawing a line connecting the medians in the boxes.

There are other ways to imply an increasing trend. You can increase the size of dots or give them a darker shading. Although it might be difficult to clearly distinguish the rank order of two values that are close together, that may not be necessary for the specific story you are trying to tell.

Going up on the vertical axis implies increasing magnitude, but it is important to have a clear and consistent reference for the axis values. Most graphing programs will automatically select a scale that extends across the range of the plotted data. This can emphasize differences between groups in your data, but it can also over-emphasize if the difference is actually negligible. It is not cheating to tweak axes to make the plot more readable, but you want to be sure that the reader understands what you're doing and why. Similarly, it is often practical to assign a common black to all graphical elements (lines, markers, etc.) except the items you want the reader to focus on, and use color or other changes to make the data of interest stand out.

Remember that white space can be your friend. Pushing numbers or graphic elements too close together will result in a graph or table that is confusing to read. The white space contributes visual variation that can improve both the readability and the aesthetics of the result.

On that note, using formatting such as alternating shaded and unshaded bands can make a table more readable, but the shading itself may not carry information. You could shade only specific rows, columns, or cells containing results you want to highlight. For a table such as demographics or model parameters, where you might have categories of different types (age brackets, BMI categories, etc.) and then shading different variables in an alternating pattern might increase readability. However, these are only suggestions and of course the journal's own requirements for formatting and layout take precedence.

We will end this section with two suggested elements to avoid. One is the "merged" cell, which allows you to define a header that distinguishes multiple rows or columns. Journals tend to prefer subheadings instead. Another is the ability to draw a 3D plot, which is just a 2D plot with depth and rotation. Such plots can be difficult to read, and the added "depth" is essentially cluttered.

CHAPTER 16

Further Reading

THIS BOOK WAS PARTLY inspired by J.W. Foreman's *Data Smart* and has a similar trick. Foreman shows the reader how to apply sophisticated methods in Excel and ends by recommending R for serious analysis work. In the prior chapters, we discussed how statistical analyses have been done and how tools could be applied. Now, we will end by describing how to view studies going forward as a researcher.

What distinguishes a statistical approach from a "data science" or "machine learning" approach may be that we assume an underlying mathematical model, an equation, or a set of equations that describe how predictors influence outcome. Then, we want to estimate the parameters and determine whether the parameters will result in a meaningful effect on the outcome.

Machine learning practitioners can argue that an explicit, intuitive model just gets in the way. Such models are inevitably wrong in some areas, and, in fact, ensemble methods in machine learning exploit this by generating many models, each expected to be wrong in a different way and taking a consensus. With modern algorithms, the computer can generate highly sophisticated models, which might not be intuitive to a human but would have improved results in prediction and classification.

We would not dismiss these approaches and, in fact, have used random forests as a way to identify a useful subset of predictors in prior studies. We would recommend Cathy O'Neil's *Weapons of Math Destruction* [60] for an in-depth discussion of the risks of an opaque model but would also recommend Frank Harrell's suggestion from *Regression Modeling Strategies* [29] that the output of a highly sophisticated machine learning or otherwise complex model could be approximated by a more intuitive set of equations, having it both ways.

We would argue for model-based studies. Our internal models are how we make sense of the world. Updating them is how we learn, going back to John Tukey's quote about approximate questions. Another relevant statistical quote is George Box's famous line that "All models are wrong but some are useful." Tukey would point out that being wrong is how the model becomes useful. Perhaps the parameter estimates will be unrealistic. Perhaps the model predictions will be nonsensical. Perhaps the difference between real data and the model's prediction indicates that the model is systematically making worse predictions in certain cases. Perhaps a reader, ideally a reviewer prior to publication, may see a flaw in the model assumptions, and perhaps another researcher publishes an alternative model that explains the data just as well.

No statistical approach should ever substitute for thought or be applied without consideration of the interpretation and credibility of the results. If the model is a poor fit for the data, then ask how the model could be improved. If an alternative model works just as well, ask what differences between models could be used to determine which one was a better representation. The back and forth between theoretical models and practical facts is how learning takes place. Even a clearly wrong model may still be practically useful. Newtonian physics is the wrong model at the scale of relativity or quantum mechanics but is very useful on the scale where most of us function. The trick is to be selectively wrong, and not (also quoting Box) "to be concerned about mice when there are tigers abroad."

We began this book by asking if it were possible to predict the future. The only prediction we will risk here is that learning never stops. Research papers are rarely definitive, and Dr. Maltenfort is always acquiring new statistics texts to the ongoing consternation of his wife.

Statisticians and machine learning practitioners both agree on the importance of exploratory data analysis. Exploration is not just a matter of checking for outliers. You may want to test assumptions, look for unexpected relationships, or check for values of predictors or outcomes that are so rare that it might be worth excluding them or combining them with other categories. For a statistician, exploratory data analysis might determine whether it is necessary to account for relationships that may not be strictly proportional or may be dependent on the presence of another factor, requiring transformations or interaction terms. For a machine learning specialist, exploration of the data makes it possible to plan for issues that may affect algorithm performance.

There is another point where statisticians and machine learning practitioners generally agree: the "no free lunch" theorem. Although some methods may become familiar and trustworthy for researchers working in a particular area, there are no approaches that are automatically best across all circumstances. As with planning surgery for an individual patient, designing an individual study must consider the particular needs and issues specific to the situation.

Clifford Stoll, who has written on a number of computer topics, has been quoted as saying, "Data is not information, information is not knowledge, knowledge is not understanding, understanding is not wisdom." Ideally, applying proper analysis turns data into information. New information is judged against existing information and vice versa, and a manuscript is written to share knowledge. Read many articles and consider what they have to say – and what they don't say, can't say, or perhaps shouldn't have said– and you develop understanding. Each of us has to acquire wisdom independently.

Glossary

Glossary: A simplified dictionary. Very unlikely to actually be glossy, although complex concepts may be glossed over airily.

In this case, the product of someone who has read both statistical texts and Ambrose Bierce's "The Devil's Dictionary." The latter is available online and is recommended to anyone with excessive optimism that diligence and data acquisition can solve any problem.

Statistic: The distillation of a set of data into a single number, hopefully useful. This may be a *descriptive* statistic which tells you something about a single measured quantity or a *test* statistic which tells you whether two quantities covary in a way inconsistent with random chance.

Inappropriately applied to the corpse du jour in police dramas; the proper terms in this case would be data point, datum, or cadaver.

Probability: That fraction of all possible events where the observed events will meet a specified condition (gender is female, age is less than 20, etc.). Since it is very impractical to do this for the entire population, it is usually estimated from an accessible sample, which is, hopefully, also a representative sample.

Conditional probability: The probability of an event happening, given that another event has been observed. The notation is p(A|B), which is read "the probability of A given that B was observed."

It is not actually required that B *precedes* A. We could ask whether it is true that the patient has a condition given that they tested positive or that they test positive given that they have the condition.

Mean (or average): Unintentionally pejorative terms which refer specifically to a descriptive statistic:: what value for a continuous variable (age, height, weight, etc.) is most representative of the entire population?

The most common one is the arithmetic mean. Next most familiar is the median. There are also the geometric mean, the harmonic mean, and the median. Each of these has different advantages for different kinds of data; for example, the median is relatively immune to extreme values, while the harmonic mean is useful in cases where it is necessary to weight the smallest value.

Standard deviation (variance): Different ways of summarizing the spread between the arithmetic mean and the measurements it was calculated from. The standard deviation is the square root of the variance in the same units as the mean, and we can speak of value being so many standard deviations from the mean. The variance is the term directly used in statistical calculations such as regressions.

Squares and square roots force variance and standard deviation to be positive even when differences from the mean may be positive or negative. It is possible to use the mean of the absolute value of the difference or even median of the absolute value, but this sacrifices computational simplicity for no real improvement in understanding.

Distribution: The mathematical description of the probability of a variable having a specific value when observed. For all possible values of the variable, the summed distribution must be 100%, and no probabilities can be negative.

Familiar probability distributions are the Gaussian, binomial, and Poisson. The capitalization is because there is no one named "binom" although a data made up only of zeroes and ones is called a Bernoulli distribution.

Gaussian distribution: The specific bell-shaped distribution most commonly assumed in statistical tests. Also called the normal distribution. It can be shown mathematically (the central limit theorem) that the Gaussian distribution can arise from the sum of other random variables, which may not themselves be Gaussian. Whether the Gaussian distribution is truly normal or merely traditional, it is certainly convenient: it is completely defined by the mean and the standard deviation, and knowing both allows us to make statements about the probability of observations having certain values or ranges of values.

Regression: In an individual, the return to a less mature, developed, or sophisticated phase.

In statistics, a popular and generally useful tool for estimating how outcomes may depend on predictors. The tool takes its name from "regression to the mean," which is the observation that if a random variable has an extreme value when measured, the next measurement will tend to be less extreme, that is closer to the mean.

Regression comes in many flavors, depending on the nature of the outcome and the statistical question at hand. A familiar type is a logistic regression which maps estimated probability to predictors.

Statistical software: An accessible method for committing statistical analyses. A few powerful packages are free, and many others are reasonably priced. Each comes with varying degrees of documentation. None comes with any mechanism of blocking inaccurately done or interpreted statistics.

An element that statistical analyses and software have in common is the principle that they are never truly finished, merely allowed to escape.

Statistical review: An assessment, preferably concise and blunt, of whether a statistical analysis is sensible, appropriate, properly interpreted, and applicable to the problem of interest. This should ideally be performed before a manuscript is sent out. It may still be usefully administered by reviewers at the journal upon the submission of the manuscript, but don't rely on it.

Estimate: A guess that has presumably been thoroughly and properly educated by the available data. Like animals, safe to handle as long as the appropriate margins of error are respected.

Expert: A scholar of mistakes, whose existence is justified by preventing others from committing them. Experts whose education is primarily or exclusively the mistakes of those other than themselves should be regarded with appropriate precautions and from a respectful distance.

References

1. Biostatistics for Biomedical Research: Vanderbilt Institute for Clinical and Translational Research. Available from: https://hbiostat.org/bbr/.
2. Abelson RP. *Statistics as Principled Argument*. New York: Taylor & Francis; 1995.
3. Stigler SM. *The Seven Pillars of Statistical Wisdom*. Cambridge, MA: Harvard University Press; 2016.
4. Reinhart A. *Statistics Done Wrong: the Woefully Complete Guide*. San Francisco, CA: No Starch Press; 2015. Available from: https://www.statisticsdonewrong.com/index.html.
5. Huff D. *How to Lie with Statistics*. New York: WW Norton; 1993.
6. Good PI, Hardin JW. *Common Errors in Statistics (and How to Avoid Them)*. 4th ed., Wiley; 2012. Hoboken NJ.
7. Tukey JW. The future of data analysis. *Ann Math Stat*. 1962;33(1):1–67. doi:10.1214/aoms/1177704711.
8. Tukey JW. Sunset Salvo. *Am Stat*. 1986;40(1):72–6.
9. Foreman JW. *Data Smart: Using Data Science to Transform Information into Insight*; 2014. Wiley, Hoboken NJ.
10. Harrell FE. Classification vs. Prediction 2019. Available from: https://www.fharrell.com/post/classification/.
11. Altman DG, Bland JM. Absence of evidence is not evidence of absence. *BMJ*. 1995;311(7003):485. Epub 1995/08/19. doi: 10.1136/bmj.311.7003.485. PubMed PMID: 7647644; PubMed Central PMCID: PMC2550545.
12. Altman DG, Bland JM. Statistics notes: the normal distribution. *BMJ*. 1995;310(6975):298. Epub 1995/02/04. doi: 10.1136/bmj.310.6975.298. PubMed PMID: 7866172; PubMed Central PMCID: PMC2548695.

13. Perezgonzalez JD. Fisher, Neyman-Pearson or NHST? A tutorial for teaching data testing. *Frontiers in Psychology*. 2015;6:223. Epub 2015/03/19. doi: 10.3389/fpsyg.2015.00223. PubMed PMID: 25784889; PubMed Central PMCID: PMC4347431.

14. Lehmann EL. The Fisher, Neyman-Pearson theories of testing hypotheses: one theory or two? *J Am Stat Assoc*. 1993;88(424):1242–9.

15. Wasserstein RL, Lasar, NA. The ASA's statement on p-Values: context, process, and purpose. *Am Stat*. 2016;70(2):129–33. doi: https://doi.org/10.1080/00031305.2016.1154108.

16. Madigan D, Ryan PB, Schuemie M, Stang PE, Overhage JM, Hartzema AG, et al. Evaluating the impact of database heterogeneity on observational study results. Am J Epidem. 2013;178(4): 645–51. Epub 2013/05/08. doi: 10.1093/aje/kwt010. PubMed PMID: 23648805; PubMed Central PMCID: PMC373 6754.

17. Ioannidis JP. Why most published research findings are false. *PLoS Med*. 2005;2(8):e124. Epub 2005/08/03. doi: 10.1371/journal.pmed.0020124. PubMed PMID: 16060722; PubMed Central PMCID: PMC1182327.

18. Ioannidis JP. How to make more published research true. *PLoS Med*. 2014;11(10):e1001747. Epub 2014/10/22. doi: 10.1371/journal.pmed.1001747. PubMed PMID: 25334033; PubMed Central PMCID: PMC4204808.

19. Gelman A, Loken E. The statistical crisis in science. *American Scientist*. 2014;102(6):460–5.

20. Halsey LG, Curran-Everett D, Vowler SL, Drummond GB. The fickle P value generates irreproducible results. *Nat Methods*. 2015;12:179–85.

21. Walker E, Nowacki AS. Understanding equivalence and non-inferiority testing. *J Gen Intern Med*. 2011;26(2):192–6. Epub 2010/09/22. doi: 10.1007/s11606-010-1513-8. PubMed PMID: 20857339; PubMed Central PMCID: PMC3019319.

22. Altman DG, Bland JM. How to obtain the confidence interval from a P value. *BMJ*. 2011;343:d2090. Epub 2011/08/10. doi: 10.1136/bmj.d2090. PubMed PMID: 21824904.

23. Altman DG, Bland JM. How to obtain the P value from a confidence interval. *BMJ*. 2011;343:d2304. Epub 2011/01/01. doi: 10.1136/bmj.d2304. PubMed PMID: 22803193.

24. Cohen J. A power primer. *Psychol Bull*. 1992;112(1):155–9. Epub 1992/07/01. PubMed PMID: 19565683.

25. Cohen J. *Statistical Power Analysis for the Behavioral Sciences.* New York; London: Psychology Press; 2009.
26. Norman GR, Sloan JA, Wyrwich KW. Interpretation of changes in health-related quality of life: the remarkable universality of half a standard deviation. *Med Care.* 2003;41(5):582–92. Epub 2003/04/30. doi: 10.1097/01.MLR.0000062554.74615.4C. PubMed PMID: 12719681.
27. van Belle G. *Statistical Rules of Thumb.* 2nd ed.Wiley; 2008.
28. Bland JM, Altman DG. Correlation in restricted ranges of data. *BMJ.* 2011;342:d556. Epub 2011/03/15. doi: 10.1136/bmj.d556. PubMed PMID: 21398359.
29. Harrell F. *Regression Modeling Stratgies: With Applications To Linear Models, Logistic And Ordinal Regression, And Survival Analysis.* Place of publication not identified: Springer; 2016.
30. Riley RD, Ensor J, Snell KIE, Harrell FE, Jr., Martin GP, Reitsma JB, et al. Calculating the sample size required for developing a clinical prediction model. *BMJ.* 2020;368:m441. Epub 2020/03/20. doi: 10.1136/bmj.m441. PubMed PMID: 32188600.
31. Charig CR, Webb DR, Payne SR, Wickham JE. Comparison of treatment of renal calculi by open surgery, percutaneous nephrolithotomy, and extracorporeal shockwave lithotripsy. *Br Med J (Clin Res Ed).* 1986;292(6524):879–82. Epub 1986/03/29. doi: 10.1136/bmj.292.6524.879. PubMed PMID: 3083922; PubMed Central PMCID: PMC1339981.
32. Wickham H. Tidy Data. *J Stat Soft.* 2014;59(10). doi: 10.18637/jss.v059.i10.
33. Altman DG, Royston P. The cost of dichotomising continuous variables. *BMJ.* 2006;332(7549):1080. Epub 2006/05/06. doi: 10.1136/bmj.332.7549.1080. PubMed PMID: 16675816; PubMed Central PMCID: PMC1458573.
34. Giannoni A, Baruah R, Leong T, Rehman MB, Pastormerlo LE, Harrell FE, et al. Do optimal prognostic thresholds in continuous physiological variables really exist? Analysis of origin of apparent thresholds, with systematic review for peak oxygen consumption, ejection fraction and BNP. *PLoS One.* 2014;9(1):e81699. Epub 2014/01/30. doi: 10.1371/journal.pone.0081699. PubMed PMID: 24475020; PubMed Central PMCID: PMC3903471.
35. Jaramillo S, Montane-Muntane M, Capitan D, Aguilar F, Vilaseca A, Blasi A, et al. Agreement of surgical blood loss estimation methods. *Transfusion.* 2019;59(2):508–15. Epub 2018/11/30. doi: 10.1111/trf.15052. PubMed PMID: 30488961.

36. Charlson ME, Pompei P, Ales KL, MacKenzie CR. A new method of classifying prognostic comorbidity in longitudinal studies: development and validation. *J Chronic Dis*. 1987;40(5):373–83. Epub 1987/01/01. doi: 10.1016/0021-9681(87)90171-8. PubMed PMID: 3558716.

37. Deyo RA, Cherkin DC, Ciol MA. Adapting a clinical comorbidity index for use with ICD-9-CM administrative databases. *J Clin Epidemiol*. 1992;45(6):613–9. Epub 1992/06/01. doi: 10.1016/0895-4356(92)90133-8. PubMed PMID: 1607900.

38. Quan H, Sundararajan V, Halfon P, Fong A, Burnand B, Luthi JC, et al. Coding algorithms for defining comorbidities in ICD-9-CM and ICD-10 administrative data. *Med Care*. 2005;43(11):1130–9. Epub 2005/10/15. doi: 10.1097/01.mlr.0000182534.19832.83. PubMed PMID: 16224307.

39. Quan H, Li B, Couris CM, Fushimi K, Graham P, Hider P, et al. Updating and validating the Charlson comorbidity index and score for risk adjustment in hospital discharge abstracts using data from 6 countries. *Am J Epidemiol*. 2011;173(6):676–82. Epub 2011/02/19. doi: 10.1093/aje/kwq433. PubMed PMID: 2133 0339.

40. Wright A, Hannon J, Hegedus EJ, Kavchak AE. Clinimetrics corner: a closer look at the minimal clinically important difference (MCID). *J Man Manip Ther*. 2012;20(3):160–6. Epub 2013/08/02. doi: 10.1179/2042618612Y.0000000001. PubMed PMID: 23904756; PubMed Central PMCID: PMC3419574.

41. Maltenfort M, Diaz-Ledezma C. Statistics in brief: minimum clinically important difference-availability of reliable estimates. *Clin Orthop Relat Res*. 2017;475(4):933–46. Epub 2017/01/05. doi: 10.1007/s11999-016-5204-6. PubMed PMID: 28050812; PubMed Central PMCID: PMC5339150.

42. Kronmal RA. Spurious correlation and the fallacy of the ratio standard revisited. *J Royal Stat Soc Series A (Stat Soc)*. 1993;156(3):379–92.

43. Steyerberg EW. *Clinical Prediction Models*. 2nd ed. Switzerland: Springer; 2019.

44. Parvizi J, Huang R, Raphael IJ, Arnold WV, Rothman RH. Symptomatic pulmonary embolus after joint arthroplasty: stratification of risk factors. *Clin Orthop Relat Res*. 2014;472(3):903–12. Epub 2013/11/23. doi: 10.1007/s11999-013-3358-z. PubMed PMID: 24264881; PubMed Central PMCID: PMC391633.

45. Parvizi J, Huang R, Rezapoor M, Bagheri B, Maltenfort MG. Individualized risk model for venous thromboembolism after total joint arthroplasty. *J Arthroplasty.* 2016;31(9 Suppl):180–6. Epub 2016/04/21. doi: 10.1016/j.arth.2016.02.077. PubMed PMID: 27094244.

46. Nunez E, Steyerberg EW, Nunez J. Regression modeling strategies. *Rev Esp Cardiol.* 2011;64(6):501–7. Epub 2011/05/03. doi: 10.1016/j.recesp.2011.01.019. PubMed PMID: 21531065.

47. Elixhauser A, Steiner C, Harris DR, Coffey RM. Comorbidity measures for use with administrative data. *Med Care.* 1998;36(1):8–27. Epub 1998/02/07. doi: 10.1097/00005650-199801000-00004. PubMed PMID: 9431328.

48. van Walraven C, Austin PC, Jennings A, Quan H, Forster AJ. A modification of the Elixhauser comorbidity measures into a point system for hospital death using administrative data. *Med Care.* 2009;47(6):626–33. Epub 2009/05/13. doi: 10.1097/MLR.0b013e31819432e5. PubMed PMID: 19433995.

49. Gary King, and Richard Nielsen. 2019. "Why Propensity Scores Should Not Be Used for Matching". Political Analysis, 27, 4. Copy at https://j.mp/2ovYGsW.

50. Pearl J. Lord's paradox revisited – (Oh Lord! Kumbaya!). *J Causal Inference.* 2016;4(2). DOI: https://doi.org/10.1515/jci-2016-0021 | Published online: 13 Oct 2016.

51. Harrell FE. How Should Change Be Measured? 2019 [updated 16 Mar 2019]. Available from: http://biostat.mc.vanderbilt.edu/wiki/Main/MeasureChange.

52. Harrell FE. Statistical Errors in the Medical Literature 2019. Available from: https://www.fharrell.com/post/errmed/#change.

53. Hollis S, Campbell F. What is meant by intention to treat analysis? Survey of published randomised controlled trials. *BMJ.* 1999;319(7211):670–4. Epub 1999/09/10. doi: 10.1136/bmj.319.7211.670. PubMed PMID: 10480822; PubMed Central PMCID: PMC28218.

54. Miller JE, editor Interpreting the substantive significance of multivariate regression coefficients. *Proceedings of the American Statistical Association,* Statistical Education Section; 2008.

55. Paulos JA. *Innumeracy: Mathematical Illiteracy and Its Consequences.* New York: Vintage Books; 1988.

56. Miller JE. *The Chicago Guide to Writing about Numbers.* 2nd ed. Chicago: University of Chicago Press; 2015.

57. Miller JE. *The Chicago Guide to Writing about Multivariate Analysis.* 2nd ed. Chicago: University of Chicago Press; 2005.

58. Tufte ER. *The Visual Display of Quantitative Information*: Graphics Press; 2001.
59. Knaflic CN. *Storytelling with Data: A Data Visualization Guide for Business Professionals.* Wiley; 2015.
60. O'Neil C. *Weapons of Math Destruction: How Big Data Increases Inequality and Threatens Democracy.* London: Penguin Books; Crown Books NYC; 2018.

Index

A

Akaike Information Criterion, 88
American Statistical Association, 33
ANOVA, 43, 62
Anscombe's quartet, 86, 91–92
Arithmetic mean, 49

B

Backward stepwise regression, 87
Bar plot, 49, 119
Bayes' theorem, 13, 64–65
Bias-variance trade-off, 85
Binary variables, 25, 49, 71, 98
Bootstrapping, 27
Box-and-whisker, 48; *see also*
            Boxplot
Box-Cox transformation tool, 56
Boxplot, 48, 119

C

Categorize/not to categorize, 71–73
CCI, *see* Charlson Comorbidity
            Index
Central limit theorem, 15
Charlson Comorbidity Index (CCI),
            77
Chi-squared test, 61
Cochrane Collaboration, 45

Collinearity, 90
Confidence interval (CI), 8, 16, 22,
            36–38, 41, 45, 49, 65, 115,
            118
Correlation coefficient, 91, 105–106
Cox proportional hazards model, 77
Cumulative distribution function,
            15–16; *see also* Probability
Cumulative normal distribution, 23

D

Difference-in-difference methods, 95

E

Effect size, 40
Extreme values, 57–60

F

False-positive rate, 64
Frequentist *vs.* Bayesian, 66

G

G*Power3 software, 44
Gambler's fallacy, 24; *see also* Law of
            averages
Gaussian assumption, 30

Gaussian/normal distribution, 14–15
Generalized linear mixed model
  (GLMM), 106
Generalized linear model (GLM), 98
GLMM, *see* Generalized linear
  mixed model
Goodhart's Law, 32
Graphs, 47–48, 50, 58, 68, 79, 83, 91,
  111–112, 116, 118–119

H

Holm-Bonferroni adjustment, 42

I

Imputation algorithm, 108
Intention to treat analysis, 109
Interaction terms, 84–85
Intercept, 114
Interquartile range, 49
Intraclass correlation coefficient, 105

L

Law of averages, 24
Law of large numbers, 22
Linear regression coefficients, 115
Logarithmic transform, 56, 58
Log axes, 59
Logistic regression, 97–100
Lognormal distribution, 16–17, 48
Long-format file, 70
Longitudinal data, 70
"Lord's Paradox" question, 102, 105

M

MAR, *see* Missing at random
Matching and stratification, 83
MCAR, *see* Missing completely at
  random

Mean (or average), 58
Measurement error, 91
Median, 57
Meta-analysis, 103–104
Minimal clinically important
  difference, 78–79
Missing at random (MAR), 107
Missing completely at random
  (MCAR), 107
Missing not at random (MNAR), 107
Mixed-effects model, 104
MNAR, *see* Missing not at random
Model parameter, 84
Mortality, 77–78
Multiple imputation, 108
Multiple predictors, 83–93, 113
Multivariable models, 83–85

N

Negative binomial distribution,
  98–99
Non-Gaussian distributions, 55–57
Non-parametric test, 7, 60–61
Null hypothesis, 29–30, 32–33, 40,
  63, 65
  significance testing, 31

O

Odds ratios, 99
Omnibus test, 43
One-tailed test, 15, 41–42
Ordinal data, 60–62
Overdispersion, 99

P

Paired t-tests, 102
Parametric tests, 61
Permutation test, 32
Pie charts, 49

Poisson distribution, 58, 98–99
Post-hoc analysis, 44
Power analysis, 45
Predictor
    controlling for, 84
    effects, 84
    selection method, 89
Printed documents, 112
Probability
    ancient Greek line, sense of, 12
    Bayesian vs. frequentist view,
        12–13
Propensity scores, 93–94
Pseudoreplication, 102
p-values, 29–33

R

R®, 6
Random
    assignment, 81
    data, 12
    effects, 104
    error, 14
Receiver operating characteristic
        (ROC) curve, 78
Regression
    fallacy, 26
    imputation, 108
    to the mean, 26
    slope, 44
Regression Modeling Strategies
        (Frank Harrell), 122
Residual plot, 91
Risk ratio, 38, 99

S

Sample size, 44
    vs. p-value, 35–36
Sensitivity, 5, 64
Sharp null hypothesis, 29–30

Significance test, 33, 65
Simpson's paradox, 50
Skewed distribution, 16, 49, 55, 69,
        91, 98
Spline, 72
Spurious correlations website, 34
Standard deviation (SD), 7, 14, 21
Standard error (SE), 17, 27, 65
Statistical analysis
    application and presentation
        of, 4
    goal, 13
    methods, 95
    principles of, 5
Statistical estimates, 25
Statistical tests, basics of
    confidence interval (CI), 36–37
    productivity, perils of,
        33–34
    p-values, 29–33
    sample size *vs.* p-value, 35–36
Statistics, language of, 22
Statistics as Principled Argument
        (Robert Abelson), 4, 112
Stepwise regression strategies, 87
Story articulation, 117–118
Straight-line regression, 26

T

Table, 48
    vs. graphs, 116–117
t-distribution, 27
Test statistic, 29
Treatment *vs.* outcome, 71
t-test/regression, 30, 40
Tufte, Edward, 51, 118
Tukey, John, 5–6, 47, 76, 122
Two-tailed t-test, 41
Type I error, 31, 41
Type II error, 31, 41
Type III error, 32

U

Underdispersion, 99
Underfitting *vs.* overfitting, 85–86
Unpaired t-tests, 102

V

Valid inferences, 26
Variance inflation factor, 90
Visual lingo, 118–120

Printed in the United States
By Bookmasters